This Book Won't Cure Your Cancer

GIDEON BURROWS

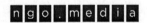

ngo.media

Whatever this is...

I DON'T REMEMBER telling my wife I had a deadly brain tumour. I do remember watching my family doctor walking up the driveway to our little bungalow. It was sunny and Erin and Reid were playing in the garden. I was watching them through the window as they picked leaves, twigs and flowers, building a nest for their toys to sit in. We lived in a tiny village, so it didn't seem strange at all to see our local doctor walking up our drive to make a house call.

I remember his shoes. They were patent black and well polished. He kept them on and refused a cup of tea. The children ran in and out of the house with daisies for him, which he patiently lined up on the arm of the sofa. It was Monday morning and I'd had an MRI scan the Friday before. He asked how all the tests had gone and I told him just fine. It was only when he was about to leave that he said what he'd really come to say. Looking back, it must have taken some courage.

"I need to tell you that I've had some news. It's a bit difficult with the children around, but the MRI scan found something." I nodded. I could feel my heart beating in my chest. I was wearing my 'Eat, Sleep, Cycle' T-shirt. "A lesion," he said.

He knew little more. I was to go to a hospital to see a specialist. A brain surgeon. He'd already made me an appointment for Thursday. He handed me the note for the meeting. "I've already written you a prescription for some steroids. And," he hesitated, "I have to ask you not to drive. At least until you've seen him." He asked me where my wife was. I said I'd call her at work and ask her to come home.

My doctor never actually said the words. He didn't need to. It all hung in the air so obviously between us that it didn't need to be uttered. We shook hands and I thanked him, just as if he'd popped in for a friendly visit. I watched as he dragged those polished black shoes back down the driveway, his head hanging low. He waved to the kids as they went about their games.

I called them in. Erin was just gone four, her brother Reid barely two. How could they understand? I knelt on the rug in our living room and asked them for a hug. They indulged me for 30 seconds, no more. Even as they struggled to get away, I buried my face in their hair and desperately inhaled the smell of them. Shampoo. Mown grass. Sun cream. Eventually they broke free. I was left alone on my knees, staring at the floor.

I texted my wife Sarah to ask her to call me when she got out of her meeting. I then thought of my brother and when I had been living in London ten years before. I was out with some friends in a pub near the River Thames. His number flashed up on my phone for the third time that evening and I finally went outside to answer it. "I'm sick," he had said. "That lump on my collarbone has been tested. It's Hodgkin's Lymphoma. I have to start radiotherapy tomorrow, and have chemotherapy too." It was a brief conversation but when I walked back into the bar that night, I quickly made my excuses. I went home.

Still on my knees, I looked down at my phone then back up to my kids playing in the garden. I clicked through to my brother's number and he answered on the first ring. "The doctor has just been around with some test results and I'm sick," I said. "I've got a brain tumour." We spoke for a little

2

while, but there was nothing more to say. I remember the choke in both of our voices, as if we couldn't quite utter the word.

Cancer.

I don't remember tears that afternoon while I waited for my wife to return. The sky didn't fall in. I was puzzled. Amazed. So this is what cancer feels like? I tried it on like a new shirt. It felt just like the one I'd been wearing before my doctor had come. I made a cup of tea. I picked up Erin and Reid's toys and stuffed them under their beds. I thought about making dinner. I wandered around the garden and raked over the vegetable beds.

I don't remember too much about the few days that followed. I know I picked up the drugs my doctor had prescribed. My wife took video footage of me taking the first steroid pill later that afternoon. I don't know why she wanted to record it. I held the tiny white tablet up to the camera. "Here's to ... whatever this is." I swallowed the pill and raised the glass of water as if toasting the future.

I suppose we must have cried together. We must have hugged a lot. We must have spent time on the internet, looking up information about brain tumours, absorbing statistics and stories on cancer websites and charity talk-boards. We must have watched our children with wide eyes, drinking in every moment of them, knowing what people often forget. This moment, this exact sliver of time, will never come back.

Brain cancer equals death. Sure, there are a few ways to add up the sums. A few parenthesis, different methods for cutting up the numbers. But there could be little doubt about what was waiting at the end of the equation.

This book is about the first 18 months of the last years of my life. By the time you read it, there is a possibility I will be dead.

I have a very large brain tumour in the frontal lobe of the

left side of my brain. It cannot be operated on. It cannot be cured. Researchers are working hard right now to find ways to keep people with my kind of brain tumour alive for longer, but success is still far away. My death from this illness could be in another five years. Even 10, perhaps 20 if I'm lucky. But it is going to happen. That is not in doubt.

Except from day one there does seem to have been doubt. When I began telling family and friends, colleagues, clients and contacts about my inoperable, incurable brain tumour, and how it was going to one day kill me, there was lots of doubt. Actually, there was dissent. Not just the 'oh, I can't believe this is happening' and 'it just can't be true' type of dissent. There was actual, real disagreement with the facts.

A friend of a friend cured their cancer by changing their diet. There's this doctor in Canada or Germany or Ireland who does incredible things with brain tumours. I'll pray for you and ask for healing. Think positive and you'll live. Take this supplement and it'll kill off the bad cells. Mix this herb with that tree's sap and drink it five times a day. Stop eating wheat, dairy, meat, sugar. That celebrity had cancer and then it just went away overnight. Doctors aren't always right. Let's get you some experimental treatment. What about neurolinguistic programming? Watch this YouTube video. Read this article. Visit this website. Contact this charity. It's the chemo that'll kill you, not the tumour.

Don't give up.

There's always a chance.

There's always hope.

It can't do any harm.

You never know unless you try it.

Each of these suggestions was offered with love and concern. They were heartfelt responses to the statement for which there is no adequate response: 'I have cancer.' I do not blame anyone for offering their suggestions. Some were just a stab in the dark. Others truly believed their suggestions would help me. I'm grateful, however ludicrous some of them seemed. When friends and well-wishers offer a suggestion, a treatment or an approach to cancer, they're doing so because they truly care and want to help. No one should be blamed for that.

But there is a flip side. There are those in cancer circles who care less about cancer patients than they do about the money in their pockets. There are those who have built empires on selling treatments and diets that don't work. There are those that hide or misinterpret evidence of tests that have failed to prove their treatment regime works. I was to find out all about them in the months that followed.

This book isn't about the liars and cheats, however. It's about us. Patients and the people who love us. It's about how we respond to cancer. The Big C. I want to ask: why, when it comes to cancer, do people grasp for treatments and approaches that have never been shown to work?

Why do normally rational people turn to the irrational, the unproven, the wildly hopeful? Why do we allow ourselves to be engulfed by any advice or recommendation with no stronger promise than *it might just work* and *there's no harm in trying*?

This reaches far beyond alternative medicine and bogus cures. It extends into the decisions we make about our treatment, into the choices of the charities we support, into how we treat our doctors' advice. It touches on how far we trust pharmaceutical companies, on our attitude to religion, even on how much we can trust our own judgement.

Nearly four years later, my diagnosis has not left me with what I expected. It has left me asking: what's so special about cancer? Why do we behave the way we do around it? Why does cancer have a special place in our fears, and in our attitudes to medicine and treatment? Why do we *fight* and *battle* with fellow *survivors* when it comes to cancer, and why is this war-like rhetoric rarely used with other medical conditions?

Since that first visit from my family doctor I've spent time thinking not about God, but instead about the prayers that have been offered to me. I've spent time thinking about alternative therapies. But not about trying them, nor about the biological implausibility of many of them. Instead, I've thought about the logical and philosophical flaws which undermine their whole foundation.

I've spent time thinking about mainstream doctors, oncologists and the pharmaceutical industry. Not about how they're trying to trick us or kill us, or don't do enough to spot cancer, but rather how we as patients have come to see their role in maintaining and protecting our health. I've spent time thinking about why we allow ourselves to be so easily influenced, even fooled, when it comes to cancer.

Is it desperation, despair? Some kind of resignation to the inevitable? Is it even a subconscious desire to belong to some kind of club? A tribe? A cancer cult? Ultimately, I've found myself asking: why do we let emotion so often get in the way of reasoned decision making when it comes to cancer? I have found no answers to these questions. I don't think there are any clear responses. Only more questions.

What you'll read in the following pages are musings of a man with a slow-growing brain tumour. One which I know will eventually kill me. The first 18 months of the remaining years of my life have been spent contemplating what cancer does to us. Not only to our bodies, but also to our minds and to our hearts.

Follow the orange stripe

A YOUNG MAN in a doctor's waiting room is a rare sight. Women appear with seeming regularity in the doctor's waiting room. Making small talk over issues of *Country Life* and pointedly avoiding talking about the trouble that's brought them there.

With young men, if they're in the doctor's waiting room at all, you often don't need to ask them what's wrong. Many carry some physical indication of the complaint they've come in with. Perhaps they have a plaster cast on their lower leg, and you think: got to be a soccer injury, hasn't it? An arm in a sling might be a pub-night fall, or a work-related incident. A couple of stitches above the eye or an out-of-joint nose: a boxing injury if I'm feeling generous, a drunken brawl if I'm not.

It's probably why so much is made of the infamous 'man flu'. Men don't get ill so, when we do, we really go for it. The world has ended, bring out your dead. We retreat to our sickbeds with sore throats and snuffly noses, doses of Night Nurse and perhaps a little bell to call for more headache tablets. We expect our kids to sit by our bedside, quiet and meek, as if we're a dying Pope. Yet even with a colossal man flu, the doctor's is the last place we head.

When my brother told me he was worried about a lump in his neck, I told him he was being silly. He'd shown me where he felt it, but I couldn't feel anything. He was 24 and a top-class middle-distance runner. He ran for Britain and was a likely contender for the 1996 British Olympic team for Atlanta. He was one of a select few athletes who have run a mile in less than four minutes. He was skeletal. Taught skin over tight muscle and bone. Even the slightest knot of muscle was bound to feel conspicuous when there was nothing else on his wiry body, I told him. "You don't need to go to a doctor."

I actually said those words.

When younger men go to see a medic, it's most often in a van with blue lights flashing on top. The football field injury, the dumb showing off roller skate trick. The amateur cyclist who's come down with a bunch of others after a touch of wheels – embarrassingly going only at 14 miles per hour – and ended up with patches of his skin spread across the road like melted butter over toast. Half my elbow hanging off and oozing with blood.

"Can you bring some bandages?" I ask my wife when I call to ask her to pick me up and take me to A&E. What's really painful is to see the sorry state of my beautiful black and silver Cannondale, its expensive carbon fibre frame snapped at the top tube.

The thing about being a road cyclist is this: you're invariably going to crash. It's part of the deal. A leg and an armful of scars from previous crashes aren't just proof you've been riding for many years, they're worn as badges of honour. The unsightly scarring on my left elbow is testament to that crash, as is my still sensitive left shoulder which, even years later, still can't be slept on.

That crash was in March 2012. The X-rays come up clear and I'm sent on my way with stitches in my elbow, a sling to wear for a week to give my shoulder ligaments a chance to renew themselves. I manage to stay off the bike for nearly a month, but that's as much as I can stand. It's Erin's fourth birthday. The birthday cake and pizza sit like a rock in my stomach. I need to start putting in work again for the cycling season ahead. I'm not quite fit enough to get back out on the road. To be honest, I can't really put my full body weight on that injured left shoulder. But at least I can put on some pumping music, sit on my static bike and turn my legs. Loosen up the muscles and start to bring on a sweat. With my wife and kids out to see some friends, now is the perfect time.

You get carried away with these things. After a warm-up I start to do a few short 'efforts'. Fast leg spins against an easy gear, short rests in between. It's traditional groundwork for faster speeds out on the road. During the third 10-minute effort something strange happens. It feels like a quick dropping away of consciousness on the right side of my head, as if my skull there has suddenly become empty. There's a buzzing in my face, particularly in my back teeth. I can taste metal in my mouth.

I quickly unclip from the bike pedals, move forward from the saddle and stand with my feet on the floor either side of the bike frame. There's no time to get off the bike completely. I feel the right side of my face pull down, as if the muscles have become loose and lazy. A little spit dribbles from my downturned lips and the muscles in the right side of my neck begin to tic. Songs from my childhood play in my mind like mumbled faraway echoes. My right shoulder begins to tic too, the right arm lifting up and down slightly two or three times. I try to steady myself across the bike, my left hand pressed up against a wall.

And then all is still.

My body and mind piece themselves back together. The tics stop first, then the right side of my head feels like it's reforming into proper order, blocks slotting neatly into each other to build a whole. The metallic taste ebbs away and the buzzing in my teeth stops. The spiralling had lasted perhaps two minutes, certainly no more. I have been fully conscious

9

throughout. It's as if I am watching it all happening from the inside. Now I'm fully back. I shake my head to make sure. Everything in order.

I climb off the static bike and clip-clop in my cycling shoes back to the house. I strip, take a shower and lie on the bed thinking until my wife comes home. "I think it's time to go to the doctor," I tell her when she does.

By my reckoning, this experience – what my wife and I have begun to call 'episodes' because we don't really have another name for them – is the fifth time. I've started to make a note of them. This is the most severe yet.

The first episode happened in October 2011. I'm out on a ride, perhaps 50 miles. The sun is shining and it's a good run. I'm not particularly tired but am looking forward to getting home and getting fed. About a mile from home, I squirt some water from my bottle into my mouth. Suddenly I feel my teeth begin to buzz where the water connects. I start to feel dizzy and as if my right side – head, arm, leg – has become weak and empty. I pull up and leap off the bike and onto a grass verge. The buzzing shivers down my right side for about 30 seconds and my mind does somersaults. Over another half-minute the intensity ebbs away. Then I'm standing at the side of the road with my bike, wondering what the hell just happened.

At the time I have a broken and sore molar tooth. I figure I must have squirted a stream of liquid right into the tooth, which somehow hit an exposed nerve and created a full body shudder in response. Well, that was weird. But I climb back onto my bike and spin home. The experience came and went so quickly I've forgotten about it by the time I've put my bike away. I don't even bother to mention it to Sarah.

The next two episodes happen about a month later, both during the same ride with my local cycling club. Both times, it's when the pace goes up a little and I have to start working harder. First, there is our traditional sprint for a set of 30mph signs about 25 miles into the ride. I race for the line like everyone else but soon afterwards feel that weakness coming on again. I dismount and the few cyclists who haven't already passed stop to check I'm OK. That same buzzing in my broken tooth, that same dropping away of consciousness on the right-hand side. I nod, jump back on the bike and we carry on. I'm a little embarrassed because my teammates must think I've pushed myself too hard.

Towards the end of the ride, the pace quickens for another leap. I feel the same vacancy coming on again. I drop back and let the group race ahead of me. I take a minute to let it pass, climb back on and spin out the rest of the ride. This time I do tell Sarah when I get home. We both agree I really should have that broken tooth fixed. There must be an exposed nerve in there that I'm agitating. What else could it be?

A few months later I'm out on the bike again with my cycling club: this time I'm at the front with another guy. We're pushing out a sufficiently high tempo to keep everyone breathing hard. We're against a headwind, but still cranking out a good pace. Suddenly, my mind starts to drop away again and my right side goes limp.

"I'm in trouble, I need to stop," I shout across. Then, without warning, I pull across my companion to the side of the road. I force a wave of cyclists behind me to brake and swerve, accompanied by a few (fairly earned) shouts and curses. The group stops further up the road while a couple of guys come back to check on me. I stand on a grass bank trying to shake the dizziness off. They take guesses at what it could be: 'asthma attack?' 'ambulance?' 'exhaustion?' It is then I discover I cannot speak.

Actually, I can speak: but what comes out is nonsense. Words jumbled up, other things that sound like words in my head but come out as mumbles or don't come out at all. I'm stuttering and stumbling. There are looks of genuine concern on fellow cyclists' faces. Some go on to the group to tell them what's going on. Others stay with me and I manage to indicate I'm OK with a thumbs-up. We wait for a minute or two, and my words – as well as my mind – slot back into place.

"It's cool," I say, eventually climbing back onto my bike. "It's just this tooth thing. An exposed nerve. I have an appointment to get it sorted." We ease up to the waiting group and continue our ride. I don't go for the sprints that day.

The dentist looks doubtful when I tell him that this broken molar tooth is causing these weird sensations. But he's happy to remove the tooth because it is in a pretty bad way. And for a month or so after the operation, nothing happens. I declare to my cycling buddies that the tooth has been removed and normal service is resumed.

Weeks later I board a plane to Majorca, where lots of professional and amateur cyclists go for a little warm-weather training before the racing season starts. It's a successful week, putting in the miles and tackling steep climbs. On the last day, after climbing out of the heat of a post-ride sauna, I feel the right side of my mind drop away suddenly. I have to steady myself against the changing room wall. The same dizziness. The same weakness. The same metallic taste and dim childhood songs. The same inability to speak. I've ridden hundreds of miles this week with not the slightest problem. And now this?

The next week, back in England, is the crash that forces me off the bike until my daughter's birthday a month later. A full six months since my first episode.

It's not the tooth. But what is it?

When I see my doctor on the Monday following my daughter's birthday and my severe episode on the training bike, I go in with a clear self-diagnosis. "I am having," I confidently announce, "some form of ITAs. They're mini-strokes that occur in younger patients."

The doctor looks up from the notes he's been making about my episodes and spins his chair around to face me. "You mean TIAs?" he says with a friendly grin. "Transient Ischemic Attacks? I hardly think you're the profile."

I look down at my notes, a little embarrassed. Overweight. Stressed. Smoker. He's right, the fit isn't quite as strong as it seemed to be last night when I'd found TIAs on the internet.

"But I'm not going to lie to you," he says, looking again at his notes. "I'm not happy about this. I'm not happy at all." We both let the silence sit in the air for a moment. "Here's what I'm going to do. I'll refer you to the stroke clinic at the hospital but only because they'll be most efficient at getting the tests that might tell us what it is. I'll book an appointment while you have a heart test, an ECG. And a blood test." He calls his nurse over the intercom.

"What, now?" I say.

"Yes," he says. "Right now." This isn't what I expected.

In a side room the nurse shaves patches of my chest hair and attaches sticky circular pads to skin she's exposed. Then she clamps wires to the pad and plugs me into a heart monitor. This is all a bit sudden. Ten minutes ago I'd been cycling up to the doctor's surgery. At most I'd expected him to send me away with a 'let's keep a watching brief', maybe an instruction to take it easier on the bike. Now I'm naked from the waist up, hooked up to a machine monitoring my heartbeat, and a nurse in the corner is preparing a syringe to draw blood from a vein. And more tests are being booked as I lie here.

For the first time my breezy ambivalence about these episodes becomes overtaken by the tiniest inkling of fear. The doctor has said the tests would 'tell us what it is'. The jump has been made: from an 'if' to an 'it'. I am unwell. *It,* whatever *it* is, definitely exists. *It* needs to be identified. *It* will have to be dealt with.

For two weeks I hear nothing. But now I know there is an *it* I can restart my self-diagnosis. Is there any link, I wonder, between dizzy spells and exercise? Of course there is, if you overdo it. But I've had episodes when simply cycling along at a mild pace. And there was the sauna. Plus, I've been cycling like this for a decade. I've really pushed it on the bike and not had episodes too. There seems to be no consistency. I try the scientific literature, typing the combinations of the words 'stroke', 'cycling', 'TIA', 'teeth', 'nerves' into medical journal search engines.

Quite incredibly I find a scientific paper that links mild strokes with severe gum disease. There *it* was then. My broken molar tooth had been infected and that's what's causing these episodes. I send a copy of the paper's summary to my doctor. 'Is this an avenue worth exploring?' I ask, explaining the history of my broken tooth.

The next day I receive an appointment for the stroke clinic. I cycle up to the hospital the following week. Perhaps the consultant is having a bad day, but he is probably the rudest man I have ever met. He talks to me curtly, sniffs at any idea that I am having TIAs and tells me to go next door, strip to my underpants and lie on the couch. He comes in with a little rubber hammer, a few blunt needles and some cotton wool. In between talking to his colleagues in their shared native language (which I don't understand) he tests my reactions. He knocks the hammer on my knees. Asks if I can feel this pin prick, that cotton wool.

"Get dressed," he orders when he's finished. He leaves the room without an indication as to whether I should follow him once I'm clothed, or whether I should just leave the hospital. Eventually, I knock on the door between the two rooms and his tone is one of impatience: "Come on, come on. Sit down."

"You haven't had a stroke, of course." This with a smirk, as if to say: what are you even doing here? "I suppose I'll order some alternative tests."

He wants to see my blood results, he will send me for an ultrasound of the arteries in my neck, and an MRI scan of my head. I cycle home more annoyed with his treatment of me than worried about my health.

The sonographer who does the ultrasound of my neck couldn't be nicer. We watch together on the screen as he applies cold gel and then uses the machine to look at the blood and muscles at work in the arteries in my neck. All completely fine and normal.

Another day, another test. This time it's the MRI scan, and I drive up on a Friday afternoon. The waiting room is tiny and I'm asked to fill in a form confirming I don't have any tattoos, that any piercings and jewellery have been removed, and that it is unlikely that I have any shards of metal in my eyes. Magnetic Resonance Imaging (MRI) is all about very high powered magnets, so any metal could be a danger. When it is my turn, the radiographer leads me outside to a mobile MRI unit set up in the hospital car park. There are two MRI machines inside the hospital, she explains, but this is the overflow machine set up to deal with the long waiting list.

The scans will take about 20 to 30 minutes, she says once we're inside. All I have to do is lie still while the loud whirring and buzzing takes place around me. They give me earplugs to deaden some of the din. They wheel me into a large white doughnut and the MRI begins. Seven minutes later – or around that, I've been counting the seconds in my head – they wheel me out again.

"We need to take you inside and put you on another machine," the radiographer explains. "We need to put some contrast dye into your blood so the doctors can see the intensity of blood in your brain. We can't do that here because we don't have the emergency equipment we need." The atmosphere in the MRI offshoot has changed. No more small talk, just the efficient packing up of my things. I see the outline of my head on a computer screen, but one of the radiographers turns me away, mumbling almost to himself, "There's no need to look at that."

The walk back to the main hospital building with the radiographer is puzzling. We don't talk. My emotion is one of bewilderment, not of worry. If they knew they needed to do a dye-guided MRI, why didn't they put me on a machine inside the hospital in the first place? Clearly something is wrong.

Inside, I am moved straight into an MRI room, bumping someone else from the queue. The radiographers syringe a cannula, a thin plastic tube, into my arm then fill my vein with a transparent liquid that feels cold as it travels up my arm and into my shoulder. They wheel me into the machine and the scanning begins again. This time I don't bother with the counting. Instead, I lie there as the machine whirs and clicks wondering about what just happened. Like my trip to the doctors a few weeks before, it all feels a bit dramatic. After about 20 minutes the machine stops and I'm wheeled out.

"We're going to leave the cannula in," says the radiographer. "I need to check with the doctor that we've got what we need, and if he's happy I'll take it out and you can go."

I wait on a plastic chair as another guy is brought in and ushered into the MRI room. He was limping and I glimpse the radiographer propping up his knee on a cushion ready for him to be fed feet first into the machine. Despite the unexpected events, I'm still not worried about what has happened. This is me, I think. A keen cyclist. We take visits to hospital in our stride. Like that guy in there, his broken knee or whatever – he's probably a footballer. Injuries are just part of our deal. A fact of life.

I watch a man in a suit duck into the MRI control room. A minute later he ducks out again, heading on his way without looking in my direction. The radiographer comes out a minute later and tells me I can go. She painfully tears away the plaster from my hairy arm, draws out the cannula and then sticks on a wad of gauze and another plaster where the tube has been.

"OK," she says. "That's all we need. Have a good day."

When I get home, I tell Sarah about the MRI machine switch. She laughs at my paranoia: the radiographer clamming up, the aborted first scan. They would never have let me drive home if it was anything serious, would they? Just routine. Perhaps incompetent or a little strange but routine nevertheless.

Sarah and I are in a hospital reception and are told to follow the orange stripe. From the desk, we trace the many coloured stripes from the hospital entrance and off up the corridor. We are staring at the floor, watching as colours head around corners and then branch off in different directions towards different departments and different wards. Eventually, there is only orange left. After a while it comes to a stop at the door of Sahara Ward B.

It's not so much a hospital ward as a large carpeted conference room, empty except for a few chairs. There's a vending machine in the corner, and a notice board with posters and leaflets pinned to it. In a crowded, bustling hospital it feels like an empty, wasted space. Like someone had forgotten what it was for, so closed the door and left it alone. We are on time, but the consultant is running an hour late. I go to the toilet four or five times while we wait. Just to pass the time. Just to look at myself in the mirror.

The consultant and his nurse take us from our quiet space and lead us through grey square tunnels, past wards and private rooms. We're in search of a computer and a few mismatched chairs we can pull around it. In a hospital corridor we crowd around the screen. The doctor pulls up slices of my brain from his database and uses his pen to trace the outline of a white shadow covering nearly a third of the right-hand side. He explains we're actually looking at the left of my brain: the image is flipped.

"This, I think, I'm 90 percent sure," he says, "is a low grade glioma brain tumour." He scrolls through slices of my brain, up and down, showing how deep the tumour is from top to bottom. He uses a tool on the computer to draw criss-crossing bright red lines across the shadow. Five centimetres by four centimetres. He estimates another four centimetres in depth.

"These tumours are rare," he says, turning to my wife and me. "Often they can be operated on, but yours," he returns to the screen and points to areas around the shadow on my brain, "it is too close to important functions. It is beyond my own skill to remove. I don't think any surgeon would attempt it.

"And with these glioma tumours," he turns to look me in the eye. "I'm afraid, even if they are removed, they always come back." He shakes his head. "There is no cure."

I stare at the shadow and the cross-hairs he's drawn across it. I'm in wonder at the technology and numb to what it's telling us. Sarah begins to cry.

"I just wanted you to say it was treatable," she says.

"It is treatable," the nurse replies kindly after a few moments. "It's just not curable."

The doctor looks up at strangers passing us in the corridor: patients and nurses and doctors and cleaning staff. "I'll try to find us a private room," he says.

Only now? I think. *Now you've done it? Now you've told us the worst? Now you've shown us the shadow that covers a third of my brain and told us it will kill me? Only now do you offer us somewhere private?*

The consultation feels like ten minutes, but really the doctor gives us an hour of his time and his nurse more. They answer every question we can think of. He explains about the glioma type of tumour and how this kind of pre-cancer works. It is a slow-growing tumour and that, he says, is at least something. So much is unknown about my case, he can't fairly give me an estimate of my prognosis. He tells us the treatments available in my case: radiotherapy and chemotherapy. He reminds us that these are only treatments. There is no cure. My tumour is a cancer in the making, not yet malignant but bound to get there sometime.

For now he wants to do nothing. Take it slow. I will have another MRI scan in three months' time, and that will reveal how quickly the lesion is growing. He suspects it will barely grow at all in that time and that would be good news. Too much growth might indicate it was a higher-grade tumour, a malignant cancer already. No one needs to say that would be bad news.

I smile and firmly shake the doctor's hand. My wife and I thank him and his nurse for being so clear. For making so much time for us. I want to hug them both. It's as if they have somehow given us a gift, because it could have been so much worse. In cancer, the line between good and bad is often blurred. Frustratingly. Thankfully.

Five years. That is the number I get into my head as I make calculations while we walk silently out of the Sahara Ward B, following the orange stripe back to the hospital reception and then out into the open. It's a warm spring day. People are huddled around the corner from the entrance. Smoking.

How could you? I think.

I call my brother and tell him what the consultant said. I tell him five years. The conversation is short, functional, devoid of emotion. Just passing on information. But a question hangs in the air. "Do you want me to tell Mum and Dad, or are you going to do it?"

We haven't told them anything yet. The strange stroke-like episodes I'd been having. The tests. The doctor. The consultation with the brain surgeon. They know nothing. "I'll do it," I reply. "It has to be me."

I can only just hear ringing on the other end of the line. There are building works going on at the hospital, so I try to tuck myself away around the corner. Away from the noise and away from the smokers. This isn't something I want to do inside, surrounded by strangers heading this way and that, following their different coloured lines along the corridors. I don't want nurses and doctors and their patients in the lunch queue to be forced to listen in.

The ringing tone repeats and I'm hoping that my mum won't pick up. Then she'll miss the call again later, because she lives in Cyprus and there's a two-hour time difference. And maybe tomorrow too. Maybe I'll never get through. Maybe I'll never have to make this call. Maybe I'll never have to say the words.

She answers, of course. She's just come in from the garden, where she and her partner have been busy digging. They're trying to get the house ready for its first bed-and-breakfast guests.

"Hi Mum, how are you?" Pleasantries first, get them out of the way. She talks for a while, as she always does, about progress on the house. The car has broken down, which means she's had to call in a favour from a guy to bring in some sand and shift some stones about. There's someone coming in to repair the pool because it has a leak and they need to prepare it for the holiday season that's almost upon us.

I know it's not coming because it very rarely does. It's not malicious, it's just she's so used to talking about progress on her house that's she's got into the habit of not asking: so how are you? There's no choice but to stop her one-sided conversation. "Mum, where are you?" What I really mean is: are you sitting down? Are you with someone? But all that feels too harsh and cliched. Letting the bad cat out of the bad bag.

"I'm here, in the house, of course. Gez is in the kitchen getting us drinks."

"Can you call him over? I need him to be with you."

There's a muffled sound on the other end of the line and she comes back on. "OK," she says. There's a happy expectancy in her voice. A chirpy tone that says: you're obviously having another baby, but I'm not going to spoil the moment.

"Mum," I say. A drilling starts and I wish there was somewhere quieter to do this. "Mum, I'm at the local hospital. I've just come out of a consultancy with," I've gone too far now, I can't go back on this, "a brain surgeon. I've been having some tests, and he says I have a brain tumour."

I don't hear tears. I don't expect tears. I expect she's staring at the wall, more puzzled than anything else. After a moment she says: "What do you mean? What's going on?"

"Mum, the news is not good. I've only just come out. They're not sure, but they think it can't be operated on. It can't be cured." I tell her about the seizures, the month of tests that I'd kept from her. "I didn't want to tell you until we were sure. Only, I'm not sure what's going on even now."

I suddenly realise there's something thrilling about all this. It's like I'm a gossip with news to share. It's as if I'm talking about someone else. I feel a rush of adrenaline speaking such serious words, a strange exotic high.

"Do they know what's caused it? Do you have to have treatment?" Now I can hear a lump in her throat. Now I know is the time to get the very worst bit out of the way.

"There's so much we don't know. I have to come back in three months for another brain scan. But it's not going to go away. It's going to get worse." My heart starts beating faster and the thrill deepens. "I think my life expectancy is five years." Too much, I don't even know if that's accurate. "I think five to eight years."

I'm on autopilot. I feel nothing emotional about myself or the words I'm speaking aloud. I realise I've not used the word cancer. I feel cold, empty. I try to imagine my mum on the other end of the line thousands of miles away. I wonder what she's looking at, how she's sitting, what is the look on her face? But it's not with sorrow or grief that I share the news, it just feels functional. Practical. I wonder if I'm in shock or whether there's just little else to say.

She asks me how Sarah is, and I say she's just like me: we're just trying to absorb and understand, getting our heads around it all. We talk for a while. I tell her I need time to digest things and she probably does too. I ask her to tell my sister the news because she lives close to my mum and will be at work.

"Are you OK?" I say, but she doesn't answer. Ten minutes ago she was digging plants. She's probably left the hose running. Will she go back out there now and continue planting, or will she turn the hose off for the day and go for a walk along the seafront? Will she go into the bedroom, close the windows, close the shutters, crawl into bed and pull up the sheets? That's what I'd like to do right now. Any reaction will be understandable.

And that's the end of the call. I try my dad but he doesn't pick up, so I call my brother again and tell him I'll call our dad later. Will he get him to come over to his workplace, so he has someone with him when I break the news?

Sarah and I decide not to ask her parents to pick us up from hospital. Instead, we find a bus to take us the ten miles or so to their house. There, our children are waiting with their grandparents. Her folks don't know much yet either. Only that there's something in my brain and this hospital visit may be able to tell us what it is.

We sit at the front of the top deck of the 370 bus, but it's too crowded to talk. Instead, we hold hands and stare out of the window, occasionally squeezing each other's fingers, a reminder to each other that we're still there. I'm amazed to see normal life continues. Kids are still playing in the park. People in suits are hailing taxis; women trundle by with bulging shopping bags. Old people still drag trolleys behind them or crawl forward on walking frames. Shopkeepers are still filling plastic bowls with fruit to sell outside their stores. Perhaps I thought the clock might stop.

We climb off the bus and take the long route through the park. My brother calls and he has my dad with him and puts him on. I don't know how much he's been told though my brother has promised to let me break the worst of it.

"What's going on son?" The word 'son' chokes me. It's not a word he's used with me for a very long time. I start with the tests and the seizures, then explain that I have a brain tumour. Five to eight years, I say, but who knows really what's going on? "Don't say that," he says. "They can do all kinds of things these days."

"Yes, yes they can," I reply. "I'm sure you're right." I know he's not.

Unlike my mum, I already know my dad will never accept this until it actually happens. I tell him my brother will fill in the details. It occurs to me that my brother may have already provided more support for me in the space of a couple of days than I ever did when he was diagnosed with cancer. I found myself too busy to be there for him during the grind of radiotherapy, the pain and wearing away of chemotherapy afterwards. The thought sows a seed of regret in the deepest pit of my heart. I know I'll carry that regret until the last day of my life.

At Sarah's parents' house, I want my kids to run to the door. I want them to jump into my arms, to pull me down for hugs and tell me it's going to be OK. I want to hear about the day they've had, the fun they've been busy with at Granny and Pappa's. I want to hear their voices. Normal and familiar, a reminder of what they were when I left this morning. But Erin is colouring in the kitchen and she's engrossed. She doesn't even look up when we return. Reid is in the lounge playing with plastic figures and he gives a dismissive wave. They're oblivious, their own silent activities trumping the hopes of their needy parents.

Sarah's mum makes a cup of tea. That's what British people do whenever the tempo changes. It's one of the things that we're famous for. The beginning of a movie. The end of a movie. The return from shopping. The end of a board game. The beginning of a new day. The return of a family member from hospital with a tumour in their brain and five years to live.

For the third time that day, we explain what went on at the hospital. I wonder how many more times we can do this. There are more questions than we have the information to answer. Then there is silence and more tea, a slice of fruit cake. And then I need to sleep. It's three in the afternoon, but we've lived a week in half a day.

However you're supposed to feel when someone tells you that you have cancer, I don't think this is it. I'd like to say I'm anxious. I'd like to say I want to bang my fist against the wall and call out 'why me, why my kids, why my wife, why my life?' I want to shed a tear. To shout that it can't be true, that there must be something we can do. They've got it wrong. I want to feel panic and regret and grief and remorse and cheated and in pain. But all I feel is vacant and accepting. All I can muster is a gentle shrug of the shoulders, a nod of the head and a cold, impersonal: 'well, that's fair enough I suppose.'

There are things to be done. A will to write. Friends to tell. Loose ends to tie up. Insurance to sort out. Yes, that's what I'll take care of first. After my brother's cancer, I'd insisted we got a critical illness insurance to cover our mortgage. I almost punch the air in triumph at the thought. No more mortgage repayments, the house will be entirely ours. I want to call our insurers right now and tell them with a flourish just how much they owe us. I bet my life and won.

And then I feel greedy and self-satisfied and that thinking about insurance payouts is the last thing that should be on my mind right now while my soon-to-be-fatherless children play downstairs and my soon-to-be-single wife curls tight into a ball on the bed beside me.

And then for a few more hours, life is normal. We feed the kids something simple, something they like. That way there are no arguments and no ill-tempered words. I bath them as usual, then lever them into their pyjamas and read them stories like it's any other day. I kiss them goodnight, not with any extra meaning or emotion. Just the usual bedtime ruffle of hair, a peck on the forehead. Then we share a pizza with Sarah's folks. We don't talk about brain tumours or insurance policies or things to do; we just talk about everyday things. And then we go to bed, and I hold my wife tight in my arms as she cries and cries and cries. She tells me she loves me and she doesn't want to lose me, and I tell her I love her too and that somehow we'll get through this. Eventually, she drops off and I stare at the wall. I stare and I start to feel panic and regret and grief and remorse and cheated and in pain.

Anticancer

MY FIRST THOUGHTS about the strange effect cancer has on our thinking came within a few days of diagnosis. My mum sent me an email, something she forwarded from someone else. It contained two things that had me wide-eyed with wonder and shaking my head in frustration.

My mum calls herself a life coach and hypnotist. I suppose in the circles in which she moves she frequently receives all kinds of information, some much sounder and saner than others. I suspect once she had told her networks about my illness, she received all kinds of advice, all helpfully and honestly offered. I also suspect she'd already done some judicious sifting before sending me the email. I note that she topped the email with: "hope you don't think it's all bollocks, like I said before, it can't make it worse can it … I'm not in denial, nor trying to find magic cures, but if you don't look, you never see."

The first thing on the email was a link to a downloadable meditation programme called Brain Tumour Self Hypnosis. Clicking through to the product description – £6.99 for a download – the hypnosis sound file would reassure me that 'powerful warrior soldiers are preparing to fight for you against the cancerous cells in your brain – see these soldiers now growing in number – and they outnumber the cancer cells by millions to one – growing stronger and more powerful by the second …'

To be fair, the description went on to explain the download was 'not a medical or therapeutic device and is not intended to diagnose, treat, cure or prevent any medical condition or disease.' In which case, I wondered, what *was* it supposed to do?

The second thing in the email was a link to a newsletter from a therapeutic healing centre. It had been sent to my mum by a well-wisher who told her: 'remember, no disease is ever 100% fatal.' The newsletter contained some very strange things.

First was a link to a YouTube video trailing a movie called Cancer is Curable NOW! It promoted an hour of earnest documentary: how my doctors and my oncologists want me to suffer through the chemotherapy and radiotherapy they unnecessarily insist I undergo; how big pharmaceutical companies don't want to come up with a cure for disease because it would harm their profits; that governments and media worldwide conspire with them to hide the fact that cancer really is curable. NOW!

All it would take to kill off my cancer, the video concluded, is some simple changes to my diet and a fistful of supplements. The people behind Cancer is Curable NOW! offered a number of paid-for multi-step plans and information products for those with cancer, and for those who wanted to avoid it with a more 'natural' approach.

This type of video and its sentiments, I was to realise over subsequent months, are quite a feature of the cancer world. The presentation is of a dichotomy between the medieval medical establishment and a natural world of alternative treatments. In most cases, they are mutually exclusive.

The newsletter went on to claim that a 'scientific meta-analysis' is a type of research scientists do – collecting and analysing data from other researchers' scientific papers – when 'they can't be bothered to do their own research.' This was in the context of a meta-analysis of various alternative medicine solutions that had shown they don't work. This lazy, second-hand study was irrelevant, the newsletter insisted, and should be ignored.

Even from my basic biology lessons in school, I knew that a meta-analysis is not something a scientist does when they 'can't be bothered to do their own research.' In fact, a meta-analysis is one of the strongest and most comprehensive steps in presenting scientific evidence. It takes, for example, 10 different research papers published over a decade. It rates each piece of research for its quality, attempts to determine the implications of the different papers, presents an overview of all the research on a particular question, and then draws conclusions from what it has found. In other words, a meta-analysis can present stronger scientific evidence and conclusions than the 10 papers at which it looked. It is the very antithesis of lazy research that can be dismissed out of hand.

The writer of this newsletter simply did not know what he was talking about. A simple web search is enough to show a meta-analysis is not what he claimed it was. The problem is this: people read this stuff and they believe what they're told, particularly if they are desperate and looking for easy solutions. The writer of this newsletter was in a position of power that, used carelessly, could do serious damage. I was quickly discovering the world of cancer is a vulnerable place to be. It takes an act of will to resist gems of information that assume their own validity when they have nothing of the sort. That email annoyed me, and over the next weeks and months I was to receive dozens in a similar vein. I also received face-to-face recommendations about how this treatment or that alternative approach had prevented or cured cancer.

And it was me who felt bad. It began to appear that cancer is a place where you're supposed to listen to everything that anyone has to say, even if they have no training or qualifications in oncology (cancer treatment), or biology, or neuroscience, or surgery, or epidemiology (the study of populations and illness). I felt embarrassed. I felt too uncomfortable to tell my well-meaning saviours that what they were suggesting was probably rubbish.

I have been reliably informed by my neurologist and three different brain surgeons – all of whom have looked at my MRI scans and know a thing or two about brains – that my tumour is not pressing upon, indeed is located nowhere near, the part of that amazing organ in my skull that is responsible for rational thought. The tumour may make me dizzy occasionally and will kill me eventually. But it hasn't made me less questioning or more willing to accept just anything.

As a self-publishing writer, I know a thing or two about how the online retailer Amazon works when it comes to promoting and selling books. The basics are pretty simple. If a lot of people buy a particular book, that book goes up in the rankings for its category. If a lot of people positively review a book, the same happens. In short, if a book is popular, well read and well liked it hits the front page of Amazon. And that makes it more visible, creating more readers and more happy reviewers. (I know this because, like any author, I'm always hoping my books hit the front page too.)

If they're anything like me, one of the first things newly diagnosed cancer patients do after hearing the news is to go to Amazon (or pick your online bookstore) and type 'cancer' into that big white box before hitting the search icon. A whole load of cancer-related books come up. And because of Amazon's algorithms, the books to hit that first page of search results are those books relating to cancer that are most often bought and most often reviewed.

I was astounded. Well over half of the books that

appeared on the first page of results for my 'cancer' search were about alternative therapies, cancer-busting diets and special secrets – including the secrets that 'doctors don't want you to know' – when it comes to cancer. There were a few science books and a few autobiographies. But a notable number of the autobiographical books were also about rejecting mainstream medicine in favour of natural remedies. As an unscientific but telling test, I'm going to go to Amazon.co.uk right now and search for 'cancer'.

There are 15 entries on the front page. Of them, five are very clearly about alternative medicine and non-mainstream ways to prevent or deal with cancer, notably some bestsellers including: *Mum's NOT Having Chemo*; *Forbidden Cancer Cures*, *Foods to Fight Cancer*; *Beat Cancer: How to regain control of your health and your life*; and *The Royal Marsden Cancer Cookbook*. The top book is *Anticancer: A new way of life*.

Three are cancer memoirs, of which one is specifically promoting alternative treatment. There is the award-winning history of cancer, *The Emperor of All Maladies*. Then there are a few where the main direction of the book is ambiguous. But notably, in the first 15 results – the whole first page – there is only one single book, *The Biology of Cancer*, which is wholly about the science and medical treatment of cancer.

Search results will vary over time and in different countries, but experience tells me they're likely to be broadly similar. What does this list tell us? First, that people affected by cancer are looking for, buying books on and reviewing books about alternative approaches to the disease. It is clearly what readers want. People with cancer are looking for an alternative medicine solution to their problem.

Second is that when a vulnerable, desperate person who has just been diagnosed with cancer looks for *any* book to help them, what they're most likely to be presented with is cookbooks, miracle stories, alternative medicine and 'forbidden cancer cures'. Many contain no sound scientific evidence to prove their claims or that what they promote works. They offer hope to people when they need it most, but have earned no right to do so.

To be fair, the Amazon search offers a limited overview of what books are available to newly diagnosed patients. After all, an Amazon book search is a self-fulfilling cycle. More people see alternative medicine books in their search results, so more people buy alternative medicine books and that means those books stay top of the table. People read alternative medicine books, find them useful or inspiring, so they leave positive reviews, which also keeps them at the top. It's really just evidence of how damn good Amazon is at giving us what we want.

But turn to the library shelves and a similar pattern is revealed. In every library I use in the UK, in the section on cancer the books on alternative medicine and natural healing consistently outweigh those that take a mainstream approach. There is no separation in the coding system between scientific and 'natural' or alternative approaches. That leaves alternative medicine books sitting side-by-side, indeed intertwined with books that are evidence and science based. The intertwining of the alternative medicine and the science gives the impression that the two types of books have equal weight and truth. That alternative medicine is just another choice in a wide range of responses to cancer. We can pick and choose, it says. The alternative medicine books are given far greater credibility than they deserve by sharing immediate shelf space with scientifically sound books, while the science is devalued by the alternative medicine books they sit next to.

All of which would be pretty petty if it wasn't real lives we were talking about. If the newly-diagnosed, or their families, go to the library and head for the cancer shelves they should be getting true, honest and accurate information about their condition and treatments. When an alternative medicine book sits right next to a booklet from a reputable scientist or a cancer charity's guide to mainstream cancer treatments, they are presented as an equal choice for potentially saving your life. And they are not. Pick the wrong book because you like the bright pictures of fruit and leaping healthy bodies on the cover, and you could be led into an erroneous impression of your chances. Or worse, you could be led into a life-threatening decision based on iffy information.

I'm not saying alternative books on cancer should not exist. Rather that they should not sit next to scientifically evidenced books as if the two were the same thing. They should sit in 'healing', or 'alternative health' or perhaps some other category of their own to avoid confusion.

In the world of cancer, one book towers over all the rest. It is a 'must buy'. If you have cancer, or if a loved one has cancer, you have probably already heard of it. If you haven't, you soon will.

Anticancer: a new way of life by David Servan-Schreiber is the biggest cancer book of all time. No other cancer book comes close to the sales it enjoys. It has been translated into 35 languages and published in 50 countries. It has sold over one million copies. It is, as the cover exclaims, 'The Number One International Bestseller'.

I bought the book, of course, and it did have the most profound effect on me in those first early weeks. But, for me, the effect of the book was one of huge disappointment and certainly not the positive read I had expected. The book is well written and Servan-Schreiber's story is compelling. Aged 31, he was working as a doctor of psychiatry, running a lab funded by the National University of Health in Pittsburgh, USA. By using MRI scans, he and his colleagues were looking at ways to map thought in the workings of the brain. This was a guy who knew a thing about brains and biological functions.

Like many scientists do, he went under the scanner himself as part of an experiment. The plan was that he would do mental tasks while being scanned; his colleagues would watch to see which parts of his brain lit up.

The experiment is all going to plan but after 10 minutes his colleagues stop taking images. They uttered words not too dissimilar to those I heard after my own first brain scan: "Listen, there's something wrong. We're coming in." A few minutes later they broke the news: "We can't do the experiment. There's something in your brain."

He had a deadly brain tumour.

What follows in *Anticancer* is a chapter-by-chapter tale of Servan-Schreiber's post-diagnosis life including his initial surgery, but also the approach he takes to attempt to prevent the recurrence of his tumour and the future development of his cancer into something that might kill him. It starts with information about how the science works and medically sound and proven techniques for treating cancer. But after a few chapters, it begins talking with apparent authority about unproven cancer causes and remedies. Servan-Schreiber talks about eating cancer-busting foods. He introduces his core premise of cutting back on sugar, particularly certain types of sugar. He lists the most helpful fruits and vegetables, supplements and ingredients, and the less helpful ones, for beating cancer.

We learn the specifics of how certain mushrooms prevent breast cancer growth, and that herbs and spices and superfoods can prevent or block cancer. He introduces a daily anticancer diet (the anticancer plate) including green tea, turmeric and curry powder, citrus, chocolate, red wine, foods rich in selenium, garlic and specific types of fish.

He then moves on to our mental state: how staying positive, practising mindfulness, meditation and 'focusing on the self in the present' helps cancer patients to live longer. And he concludes, by the end of the book, that following this regime – known by his followers as the anticancer lifestyle – is key to why he has lived so long since his initial diagnosis.

This approach – keeping cancer at bay through mental balance and diet – the book calls improving your cancer 'terrain'. Servan-Schreiber never claims it can guarantee you will be cancer free, or that an anticancer lifestyle will cure cancer. But he is clear that improving your 'terrain' will improve your chances. Those most likely to live longer, he claims, 'along with with benefits of the conventional treatments they receive, they have somehow galvanised their natural defences. They have found harmony in this simple quartet: detoxification of carcinogenic substances, an anticancer diet, adequate physical activity, and a search for emotional peace.'

The book contains sense, for sure. His appeals to live a healthy lifestyle do indeed ring true: a healthy diet, regular exercise and a low alcohol intake do highlight known risk factors when it comes to cancer and prolonged survival. But alongside, the book shares advice that simply is not true and has never been proven. Servan-Schreiber jumps from single scientific studies and anecdotes to make wider conclusions about food we should and shouldn't eat, and mental states we should pursue.

A generally healthy diet is indeed related to a reduced risk of cancer, but no specific ingredient of his anticancer diet – not mushrooms, turmeric, cumin, seaweed or garlic – has ever been proven to have cancer-beating or preventative properties in and of themselves as some kind of superfood. That's a leap too far. Neither has there ever been any reliable, repeatable proof that positive thinking, meditation or mindfulness can prevent the progression of cancer. It might *sound* like sense, but the theory is not backed up by the collected evidence. Freakish single studies are taken as proof when a scientific meta-analysis of the data would more likely show they are the exception rather than proof.

What was most striking to me was that Servan-Schreiber tried to identify a cause for his brain cancer, particularly its relapse years after his initial brain surgery. He concluded it was because he hadn't paid attention to his 'terrain':

"Caught up in my work and the birth of my son, I was exercising less frequently. I had also dropped my passing interest in meditation, originally aroused by reading Jung. I had never fully absorbed the idea that if I'd had cancer, it was probably because something in my 'terrain' had enabled it to develop and I needed to take charge of myself to limit the risk of a relapse."

The idea of an untended 'terrain' as a cause of brain cancer or its relapse just didn't ring true. When I was diagnosed, I never asked what caused my brain tumour because all the expert scientific papers and cancer charities were very clear from the start. A simple analysis by Servan-Schreiber should have driven him to the same conclusion. There has never been a proven cause for brain tumours, nor their relapse. Not diet, not pesticides, not smoking, not mobile phones. Nothing. As far as the most informed and expert scientific researchers on brain tumours know, brain tumours just happen. There is nothing you can do to prevent them. It may be very bad luck, but it is bad luck nonetheless.

His approach seemed so erroneous in a book heralded by cancer patients as *the* book to read. It made me question every other word he wrote. Despite how well the book was written and how scientific an approach it *seemed* to take, in a stroke he'd made me question his credibility. It also made me feel the blame for my brain tumour rested with me. It must be something I'd done wrong. I hadn't looked after my 'terrain'. That made me not only disappointed, but angry.

The implication that my cancer was my own fault upset

me. That, of course, doesn't make it a reason to reject its truth. The thing was that Servan-Shreiber had no evidence or proof that it *was* my fault, my lifestyle or something else I had done. Nor the same for any other brain tumour patient. He had no right to be dishing out blame – either to himself or others.

I began looking deeper at the scientific studies on the one hand and looking at his book on the other. As sound scientifically as it was in some parts, it was merely useful in others and factually incorrect in yet more. I felt badly let down. Every day, *Anticancer* sat there at the top of the Amazon rankings, earning plaudits and not receiving even the slightest critical review. Rational thinking among its readers seemed to have disappeared. Yet my reading of the book, as a non-professional, newly diagnosed patient, had in a matter of just a few days found the book, along with the anticancer lifestyle it promoted, sadly wanting in most key areas.

Then one day, my disappointment with the whole anticancer project sank deeper. My wife brought home another book by Servan-Schreiber called *Not the last goodbye*. He wrote the book in the final months of his life. The author of *Anticancer*, the (unwitting) founder of the whole anticancer movement, had died. And he had died from brain cancer. His own approach, his own diets, his own remonstrations to think positive, meditate and be self-aware, had failed to prevent his cancer from returning yet again. It's a terribly sad tale, but made all the worse on reading *Not the last goodbye*. It is here, perhaps, that one would expect the author to acknowledge the inevitable. That brain cancer doesn't really have a cause. That superfoods and positivity can't prevent the natural progression of brain tumours.

But instead, he writes that he stood by what he had written. The problem was that he hadn't followed his own advice. He'd gone all over the world, talking about the lifestyle.

He'd got stressed. Maybe he hadn't eaten properly. He hadn't looked after his 'terrain'.

"Recently, I have not been the ideal embodiment of the anticancer lifestyle," he writes in *Not the last goodbye*.

There are still thousands of cancer patients out there trying to follow the anticancer lifestyle that hadn't worked for its founder. I couldn't help feeling uncomfortable that in his dying memoirs, Servan-Schreiber couldn't admit he may have been wrong.

I'm sure Servan-Schreiber really did believe that straying from his own path was what caused his brain cancer to come back. I'm sure he did firmly believe that following his own advice was exactly what had kept him alive for so long, rather than luck or the long-term effects of the conventional treatment he also had. But what about the thousands of readers who were – and still are – clinging with every ounce of hope to what he wrote in his book?

The second edition of *Anticancer* was published on 6 January 2011, with a new foreword by the author in which he writes: "My conviction that we can all powerfully strengthen our bodies' natural defences against cancer has been reaffirmed. As has my belief that this approach should be a part of preventing or treating cancer for everyone."

The author died the same year. On 24 July 2011, eight weeks after finishing *Not the last goodbye*. The cancer had returned 13 months earlier, this time yet more malignant than before. His cancer had returned six months *before* the second edition of *Anticancer* – along with his new foreword – was published.

The book continues to sell well and still remains top of the 'cancer' search on Amazon. Nowhere on the *Anticancer* page on its publisher's website (the same publisher as *Not the last goodbye*), nor on the Amazon page for the book, does it mention the arguably relevant fact that David Servan-Schreiber has died.

Nor that he died from the brain cancer that began his whole anticancer journey. When you read the reviews of *Anticancer* on Amazon, its readers clearly believe Servan-Schreiber is still alive. They believe his anticancer lifestyle works. They follow his recommendations.

The *Anticancer* story illustrates a sometimes unrealistic hope trumping a reasoned scientific consideration in cancer. The story led me to ask: why was *Anticancer*, as well as dozens of other books about alternative approaches to cancer, so well read (and believed in) while books of critical analysis and rational thinking taking scientific and medical approaches either don't get written, or are left to wallow at the bottom of the charts and don't make it onto the library shelves?

I feel uncomfortable writing these words. I am criticising the work of a man who has died from cancer, indeed from a brain tumour. All he was doing was trying in good faith to help others in his situation. He meant no harm. But my discomfort writing this story uncovers another vital issue: that criticising or even rationally analysing the work, motivations and conclusions of people in non-conventional cancer circles is sometimes viewed as unacceptable. Cancer is special, the proponents of any proposed remedies untouchable. Even if what they're proposing is wrong. Especially if they have cancer themselves. Even more so if they have died. *Anticancer* inspired me to ask the questions at the very core of this book. What is so special about cancer that makes us behave in this way? I don't have the answers to these questions. But in a world where, according to Cancer Research UK, one in two people will get cancer, they are legitimate and fair questions, however uncomfortable they might be to pose.

This book has been very difficult to write. Not only because it has forced me back over some difficult times in my life (and to anticipate yet more difficult ones to come) but also because I've had to wrestle with some sometimes contradictory problems. Many of those contradictions and difficulties necessarily remain because there are no clear answers.

So what is the book for?

It's a good question. If I'm carrying the message that we often act irrationally around cancer, who's going to pick that up and find it a heart-warming read? In response, I can only answer that I hope people do pick it up. I want this book to exist on the bookshelves, alongside the science books and alongside the alternative medicine books. I suppose I want it to be something else to consider if you or someone you love have been diagnosed with cancer. If you're reading around the subject, I hope you'll read these words as part of your consideration about what steps to take next.

I also hope it will encourage people to look at information they're provided with by alternative medicine, mainstream medicine, clinicians, charities, websites, talk-boards and elsewhere with just that little sharper critical eye. Because in cancer, things are nowhere near as simple as some people like to make out. It is not my business to make decisions for cancer patients. But I do hope patients will think more critically about what they're presented with and make better decisions for themselves as a result.

Joining the tribe

BEFORE I LEAVE the hospital appointment, the brain surgeon's nurse gives me a poorly photocopied leaflet about brain tumours and a prescription for epilepsy drugs: "You'll be on these for the rest of your life," she says breezily. The leaflet and the drugs are supposed to help. The drugs will help to prevent the seizures I'd been having on the bike while the leaflet will tell me more about my brain tumour.

I can't help but feel it is so permanent. I'll be on medication from now on, every morning and evening until the end. I think of an exhibit at the British Museum. The average person's medical intake is laid out on metre upon metre of white strips, a huge mix of tablets of all colours and sizes. Chemical compounds that keep the average human alive and healthy. But I'm no longer average. I picture a huge box, a shipping container perhaps. One piled full with tons of fingernail sized pills that – one by one – I will have to wash down with a swimming pool's worth of water.

The day after diagnosis, I take my first epilepsy pill. It's a drug I can't even pronounce, but it will replace the steroids my family doctor had put me on as a precaution. Over the next few days, I feel a deep tiredness, a simple inability to stay awake. I have to retreat to bed for an hour or two every day. At least, I tell myself, this is the medication. Didn't the leaflet say fatigue was a major side effect? Today, this same endless tiredness is something that still affects me every day of my life.

I read the leaflet the nurse gave me. Through the bad photocopying I can make out information about high-grade brain tumours, as well as more about benign brain tumours in children. There is very little about low-grade glioma brain tumours at all, just a paragraph that does more to confuse than enlighten. The nurse's final words echo as I sit there in front of the computer: "Don't go Googling about it, there's so much confusing information online".

Is a few paragraphs in this leaflet all I am supposed to go on? For three months until my next scan? Is this all I have to use to tell my friends what has happened, and what they can expect? So many questions have arisen since we walked out of hospital. Googling for answers is exactly what I will do.

There are brain tumour patients and cancer patients who want to know very little about their condition. Ivan Noble, a BBC writer on science and technology, wrote a very popular blog and book about his high-grade glioma brain tumour. Though writing about his experiences, he refused to hear much of the medical stuff himself. He wouldn't look at his MRI scans, he didn't want to know his life expectancy. He asked his wife to keep from him any information she discovered about his prospects at every stage of his treatment, and later towards his eventual death. It was his way of coping with the tumour which over three years ebbed and flowed. It was treated but it returned. Eventually, it enveloped him. He knew how hard it must have been for his wife to hide information from him. But it was the only way he could face the future.

But I'm different. I can do nothing but seek answers to every question. I need to fill each gap as it opens. I allow each thing I discover to let loose another dozen questions, each of which must itself be answered. In front of Google, I sit and try to think of the most appropriate way to start. And there is only one way. In at the deep end. 'Low grade glioma life expectancy'.

I have an empty file that I want to fill. I learn about how brain tumours work, particularly low-grade ones and the sub-type called gliomas. I learn what will later become my morbid catchphrase: my brain tumour is the better end of the bad ones. Low-grade glioma brain tumours, I learn, are rare compared with their high-grade relatives. Most brain cancers are those like the one that killed Ivan Noble: grade IV, almost unstoppable tumours that are as quick growing as they are malignant. High-grade gliomas are highly malignant. The larger they are, the more damaging they can be. Life expectancy from diagnosis to death could be anything up to more than five years, but it is often far less. Sometimes months. Death is certain; it is mostly just a matter of treatment. And then time.

My tumour is most likely to be a grade II tumour, a rare low-grade glioma. "I'm 90 percent sure," the surgeon had said. I may be rare, but I'm lucky to be so. When you hear on the news or read in a fundraising pamphlet that this man, that woman or that child is 'suffering from a *rare* form of cancer' you can't help but assume it's bad news to come. That they are in the final throes. In my case, those tables are turned. For me, rare means good. Rare means lucky. Rare is 'the better end of the bad ones'. Rare means go away for three months, we'll do another scan and see how your tumour is getting on. I begin to understand.

My tumour is likely to be slow growing. Sometimes low-grade tumours are very slow growing. There are a number of different types, and a group of different factors like genetics and size and position that affect them and the impact they have on the patients. Those factors also affect the length of remaining life you can expect. I drill down further. Seven years, I read in one scientific paper. Another says eight, and that's just the median: half of patients have died eight years after diagnosis, but that means half are still alive.

But with each page I read, and each scientific paper I download, there come caveats. There are contradictory generalisations and then particulars and specifics. My amateur understanding of the science and attempts to draw conclusions for my particular case leave me little the wiser. This, I know, is the nature of scientific papers. Answers are rarely clear cut, they have to be brought together in fives or tens, their individual results rinsed out and rearranged into a meta-analysis to really be meaningful. And even then, they won't predict the development of my own illness.

But a couple of phrases recur in each paper I find. They ring like bells, reminding me of what's to come. Low-grade brain tumours most often start off 'indolent': lazy, doing nothing much, harmless. But these once 'indolent' brain tumours always 'progress'. They turn into something much more aggressive, a truly volatile cancer for which there is no cure. Or they run out of space in the brain, and reduce quality of life, and then end life itself. My type of low-grade glioma may take longer to get round to it than their high-grade sisters, but death is certain. How long cannot be said.

One day I may be able to have a biopsy to pin my tumour type down a little further, to push away the confusing chaff and reveal the more accurate numbers I already crave. But a biopsy is brain surgery, and brain surgery does not come without risk. Patients with inoperable brain tumours like mine are often asked to wait, to see how things go. When the time is right, there are treatments available for low-grade gliomas. I read the too-short list. Surgery, radiotherapy, chemotherapy. But, for now, I have to wait. Three months and another scan. One day in and already it is unbearable. I crave certainty; I need to know. I can't be merely one of a bunch of statistics lumped together among others who may or may not have the same tumour that I may or may not have.

Within a week of being diagnosed and word passing around my immediate family, my sister posted information about my illness on Facebook and said she was thinking about 'my brave brother Gideon.' I immediately asked her to take it down. This might seem like a perverse reaction to your own sister reaching out as best she could. But there was so much about that post that seemed wrong to me. I couldn't at the time see the kindness she was attempting to show.

I was annoyed because she'd posted without my permission. There are no secrets on the internet. She'd announced my illness to the world before I'd even decided when I would tell even a wider group of friends, let alone work colleagues, clients and others. It was me, I told her, that had the right to decide about telling people about my brain tumour, not her. Tell the world, I said, and people I loved and wanted to tell myself would find out in an idle browsing of their Facebook feed. Looking back, what I really feared was a lack of control. Since diagnosis, I'd felt little but my life spiralling away from me. The release of the information itself was at least something I could keep a grasp on. I needed something to hold on to.

But she meant no harm. She took it down without hesitation and we left it at that. Hindsight shows me I could have been more sensitive in explaining my response. But in those first few days, I was in no state to be reasonable – even rational – about anything. That's how knee-jerk and raw our reactions to cancer can be.

But it wasn't just her posting the information itself that had bothered me. It was that she had called me 'brave'. At best, it was exactly the opposite of what I was being as the walls caved in around me. It didn't make sense. People still say I'm brave now, and I still don't get it. What is brave about getting cancer? I hadn't done anything. I hadn't encouraged it to try me as an opponent. I hadn't tried to stop it. On a Wednesday I didn't know I had a brain tumour, by lunch the next day I did. That hadn't suddenly changed me from an average bloke to a brave one. The tumour had happened to me. I was its vehicle. Otherwise, I played no part at all.

Merely having a brain tumour or cancer somehow, in the eyes of my sister and many others, had suddenly made me a fighter facing a dangerous opposition. I was determined. Battling. A survivor. I was brave.

And I wasn't.

Jumping into a river to save your child's life, that's pretty brave – but many of us would do that if we could. Working as a firefighter and running into burning buildings to rescue people you do not know, that's pretty brave too. And as John Diamond points out in his acclaimed cancer memoir *C*, somehow taking cancer from your child and putting it into your body so that you have to suffer, instead of your child, might be the ultimate in cancer bravery.

But if anything, I was the opposite of brave. My wife and I tried to maintain a tough and philosophical exterior (is that a brave thing to do?) but inside we were both falling apart. I was crumbling, crying and thinking extremely selfish thoughts about mine and my family's life. I swung from the extreme of acceptance in one minute to banging on the wall with despair in another.

None of this is meant as a criticism of those who use this kind of language. There's a herd and most of us follow it. What you do when you hear someone has cancer is to immediately react by telling them how well they're holding up, how brave they are, that in some way they've suddenly become more wonderful than they were a week ago.

Cancer is a cult. Looking back now, a firmly paid-up member, I can see it more clearly than when I first joined. To be diagnosed – even to be a close family member or friend of someone who is diagnosed – is to be rapidly inculcated into the tribe. A community with its own specific language, its expectations and conventions. After diagnosis, we ditch whatever charity we previously supported. Instead, we wear the pin badge of an organisation for people with our own particular cancer. Lung. Testicular. Blood. Brain tumours. We change our Facebook profiles to reflect it. We build an additional group of friends with the same diagnosis.

Left with a suddenly changed life, I looked around for somewhere new to pitch my flag. Somewhere to belong, because the past felt irrelevant. My brain tumour diagnosis made me feel part of something, it made me feel special. Maybe it *was* something I wanted to show off; though only when I was ready. I felt a shared identity, a small part of something much larger than me. Before, I carried the names 'father' and 'cyclist' around with me so ostentatiously that people bought me T-shirts to amplify my pomposity. Now I had 'cancer' to add to my list.

And there are indeed T-shirts and badges and hats and brooches and car stickers to declare our membership of the cancer tribe. We go to the events, we ask friends to run in marathons and swimming races and to shave their hair to raise money for the charities we support. We all fall in line.

Charities know this tendency well. A number of organisations I have worked with as a communications consultant have identified that those most likely to support them, most likely to donate or take action, are those affected by the condition they cover. It allows charities to operate more efficiently. To take a targeted rather than scatter-gun approach. There's nothing cynical about this. It's obvious. Those who are members of the tribe are those most likely to work hardest for it. It's simply good business planning.

That cancer can be a kind of cult is not a new idea. It is one explored in a seminal essay by *Harpers* magazine contributing editor Barbara Ehrenreich not long after she went through treatment for breast cancer. Immediately from diagnosis – in fact, even as she was going through early tests – she found herself surrounded by what she calls a culture of pink cancer kitsch. In the changing room of the mammogram department there were posters on the wall advertising cute breast cancer teddy bears, each sporting pink ribbons. Wherever she turned, the language of the tribe she had been forced to join was one of survivorship, fighting, battling and bravery. Cancer was the enemy, an evil to take on and win. Preferably while wearing pink.

Like for me, it was language she was profoundly uncomfortable with. Fundraising and support messages around cancer, from mainstream and less-mainstream charities, still centre on fighting and survivorship – a word that was invented by the breast cancer fundraising movement in the United States. At the time of writing, Cancer Research UK had launched a fundraising campaign which declares as its central slogan: "Cancer, we're coming to get you."

Barbara Ehrenreich posted questions on a cancer talk-board asking whether other people found the language around breast cancer inappropriate or at least off-putting. Among the responses she received she was told she needed to think more positively. She needed counselling if she even had to ask the question. The very questions, she was instructed, would bring the whole community down: she was now part of a community of cancer patients who were busy trying to survive. It was as if she had the struggle of the whole community to carry as well as her own. The implication was that by even doubting the rules of the cancer cult, she clearly didn't want to win the battle.

George Robinson, whose wife had breast cancer, also challenges this mainstream idea of survivorship in his book *The Cancer Chronicles*. Like Ehrenreich, Robinson writes of attending rallies of survivors with his wife: special events where breast cancer survivors walked around running tracks, dressed in pink, singing, whistling, hugging and celebrating their winning of the battle. One after another, each breast cancer patient took to the stage to declare their survivorship. They were applauded by the rest of the crowd like they had achieved the remarkable.

And maybe they had. But what about those who were not there? Those who had not survived? Those who had lost? Did they not deserve applause? Or had they not worked hard enough? Had they failed the cancer cult because they didn't *really* want to survive? The picture he paints of women standing up to celebrate their survival is moving, but the image also highlights flaws in our whole approach to cancer.

"Now there is a cancer culture," he writes, "and whether you had a harmless in situ carcinoma removed with a simple lumpectomy or are fighting the terminal stages of metastatic melanoma, you are called a survivor. In the first case there was nothing to survive. In the second case, there will be no survival … my thoughts were interrupted when a tall, thin woman with a chemo scarf grabbed the microphone and proclaimed: 'I am a second-time cancer survivor.' Was that really something to celebrate? That the cancer had come back again."

Like these two writers, I wonder too about our tendency to deify cancer, to almost treat it as something to celebrate. An enriching experience. An empowerment. In breast cancer, a particularly feminist empowerment. "What looks, all too often, like a positive embrace of the disease," as Ehrenreich writes.

If you are one of cancer's winners, then it's OK. You come out a better person and look at all these loving, supportive other members of the tribe. They will applaud you year after year as you survive yet another year 'clear' or 'cancer free' or 'in regression'. Or as I might put it, not yet dead.

One of Barbara Ehrenreich's correspondents did respond that there was nothing to celebrate about cancer: "I am also angry. All the money that is raised, all the smiling faces of survivors who make it sound like it is OK to have breast cancer. IT IS NOT OK!"

I agree. Cancer is not something to celebrate. It's not the foundation for something wonderful. It's not a tribe I wanted to join, or for anyone to have to. Cancer is terrible. It's awful. It's unfair, overwhelmingly indiscriminate, it's emotionally and physically draining. It's just brutal. It shouldn't be dressed up as soul enriching with pretty colours and cheers from the crowd for beating it into submission.

Cancer is not a brave battle to fight, it is a terrible disease to run away from. It is a puzzle to try to solve, something to try to keep at bay using the very best tools we have. Survival may be something to be thankful for (to your God, to your doctors, depending on your point of view). But when so many others die from cancer, how can survival be something to celebrate? There's nothing strong about trying to stare it down. It is not, in any way, OK.

When someone tells me I am fighting my brain tumour, that I am brave for simply having it, I don't feel moved or grateful. I already know I will never be a survivor. Do we tell a paraplegic to just get up and walk? That he can if he tries hard enough. He's so brave to sit there in his wheelchair, but he should aim higher. And once he overcomes his paraplegia, there's a balloon with 'survivor' written on it waiting for him. A thousand other recovered paraplegics ready to applaud him.

Yet in the cancer cult, because *some* people can be cured, we feel this language and encouragement to every cancer patient to fight for survival is fair game. Some days, thanks to my drugs, I barely wake up all day. It leaves my wife having to cancel most of her day's work to pick up my share of the childcare. Is that fighting? If further down the line I decide to protect my children's grief by refusing the radiotherapy and chemotherapy that can only prolong but not save my life, will that be me being brave? Or me giving up the battle?

If I pulled on pyjamas and went to wait for death in a darkened room would I be admirably facing my mortality? Or being a coward? Why isn't it OK for someone facing a life-limiting disease to run around the house crying and lamenting and banging his fists against the wall? Why isn't it OK to scream and collapse in a heap of despair and desperation?

Those who do die from cancer, early, quickly, painfully: didn't they put up a fight? Didn't they try hard enough? Are the survivors always the best fighters? The strongest willed?

I don't even know what fighting my condition would look like. Is writing this book fighting? Is trying to remain healthy and fit on the bicycle fighting? Is my giving up my old business, my old life and moving house to make life easier for me because I'm no longer allowed to drive fighting? Or is it giving in? When I can hardly wake and lie in bed staring at the wall, wondering about my children's future, is that a white flag? A surrender?

What would I have to do to bravely battle my condition? To refuse to fight, what would I have to stop doing? Would anyone be able to tell the difference? I've never been in a fight, but I'm pretty sure you have to choose to be in one. I don't wake every morning with tactics and plans. I don't have some solid resolve that if I have to go down then I'll go down all guns blazing. Cancer isn't some Hollywood action movie.

My wife was once told – by the representative of a brain cancer charity – that those who think positively about their cancer are more likely to live longer. This is nonsense: there is no scientific evidence for it. I'm just as likely to live or die from my brain tumour whether I wake up with a smile on my face every day or bury my head under the covers. We made a complaint to the charity. They apologised.

How long I have, and the methods by which my brain tumour will be treated, is an an ongoing and ever-changing journey. Battle is far from the right word. There's nothing here to win. It is my own orange stripe, turning in different directions at its own will. I have no choice but to follow to its inevitable destination. I'm not brave. I'm just getting on. Making the most of what I've got. Crying, and laughing, and forgetting, and remembering, and plodding and pedalling on. Like we all do, cancer or not.

The appointment is easy to book. The receptionist tells me I can pretty much come in any time on Tuesdays or Fridays. Whatever suits me. That's what happens when you're paying to see a doctor privately. My wife and I are offered coffee as we wait in the plush reception, right across the street from the NHS brain hospital where the coffee comes from a vending machine into which even the medical staff have to drop their own coins.

And the doctor is on time. He's extremely laid back and likeable, shows us to comfortable seats in a smart and unfussy office. He's wearing scrubs, which makes me think he's either just come from, or is about to go into, an operating theatre. This kind, bright-eyed guy will have his hands inside someone's brain today. Someone like me.

And then he actually says: "So, what seems to be the trouble?" Like doctors do on TV, though he must already know it's something to do with my brain since he's the brain guy. Actually he's one of the top brain tumour guys in the country. So he probably won't be too surprised to learn that the problem is this lump in my head and whether what we've been told I should do about it is correct.

He leans across the table and takes the data CD of my scans as well as the letter from my brain consultant. He loads up my scans on his screen and within a few seconds he's diagnosed me with a low-grade glioma brain tumour. He's soon scrolling through slices of my brain to get the whole picture. He gazes over the notes made by the other consultant.

"I do think you've been given good advice," he says. "This is a big tumour, but from what I can see there's no actual malignancy at the moment."

"And the other consultant," I say. "He said he didn't have the skill to operate on it?"

"Yes, I think that's true," the surgeon says. "This tumour would be far too dangerous to try to remove." He uses his pen to point to motor functions and speech areas in parts of my brain. "You need to take 95 percent out to extend life, and we wouldn't even get close to that in this position."

Far from frightening, this news comes as a relief. To have dramatic brain surgery excluded from the options strangely reassures me. It might seem odd to be glad to have a potentially life-extending choice removed, but to me it's one fewer thing to worry about. I'm almost grateful for his lifting the burden of decision.

I tell him that I'm having a little trouble with my life insurance claim. The claim forms didn't offer a tick box of a low-grade brain tumour, only a choice between 'benign' or 'malignant'. The telephone operator for the insurance company had asked, rather curtly, "Well, is the tumour benign or is it terminal?" From my reading, my tumour was neither. "Well it has to be one or the other," she'd said.

My surgeon shakes his head as if the story is a familiar one, "Oh no, there's nothing benign about these low-grade tumours at all." And again I feel justified and grateful. It's like a parallel world where good news is bad news and the bad news is good. I want to thank him for his certainty. The removal of a might-be. Knowledge is better than doubt. Knowledge can only be good, even if its content is bad. It is all I have.

"You do understand," he says, serious for a moment, "that this tumour is ultimately progressive, that it will transform." I know the language by now. And I think again how rarely the words have been used so far: that I have what will eventually become a deadly brain cancer. I tell him that I do understand. I ask him about genetics and radiotherapy and chemotherapy, and all manner of other ways to force him to tell me what my prognosis might be. But he only gives me the answer I expect.

"Every patient is an individual, and every tumour is in a different place and behaves differently, there's very little that can be surmised from just your MRI scans. A biopsy will tell us more." He tells me I will have to have a biopsy at some time if we want to know more about the tumour: its actual type, its behaviour and its genetic makeup. More of the knowledge I crave.

"But I think watch and wait is good advice," he concludes. "If surgery is not an option, then my advice would be to monitor this tumour to see what it does. It could be years before it does anything at all." So far, the epileptic seizures caused by the tumour can be just about counted on the fingers of one hand. And even then they've only happened when I've pushed it hard on the bike. Most other people with my type and size of tumour probably wouldn't even know about it yet.

We're running quickly towards the end of the 30 minutes allotted to the appointment. The doctor leans over the table and offers me some advice. The best bet, he says, is to apply for my care to be transferred to the National Hospital for Neurology and Neurosurgery, the brain hospital across the road. I can be looked after by his colleague. He specialises in brain tumour imaging and has particular interest in low-grade tumours. In other words, it's a perfect match. The consultant, he tells me, is also running a series of scientific studies on low-grade gliomas.

This hadn't occurred to me. For the first time, I realise this whole thing is wider than me. Bigger than what is going on inside my own skull. My tumour is one of a group of similar tumours in hundreds, perhaps thousands of other people in this country. There are experts in my tumour. There is a need to share my tumour so scientists and doctors can understand it better, so they can treat me and people like me. I may or may not be helped by the science and the research myself, but I can be part of it. I leave those plush offices not stunned, like I did when I left my local hospital. Instead, I feel justified in seeking another expert opinion. I still have a life to live. Some of that might offer a chance to get involved in some science, and to better understand more about how the brain and cancer works. Joining a scientific study may even offer the chance to contribute to the development of a cure in the future. Or at least to lengthen and improve the lives of people with similar tumours to me.

In a twist of coincidence, when I return home a letter from another hospital in Cambridge has arrived. My first hospital had arranged for me to get a second NHS opinion, and referred me to the brain surgery clinic there. I almost cancel the appointment. The first opinion and then my private visit to another brain surgeon have concurred with each other. Together, they have left me with some certainty and satisfaction that I'm coming to know my condition as well as I can. But the clinic in Cambridge is run by a couple of brain surgeons whose names have already stood out in the research I've done myself; one has written what I know is regarded as a definitive paper on low-grade gliomas. For my interest alone, it's worth the visit.

The appointment is in a week's time. In the days following

my London appointment I feel something change in me and my attitude to the brain tumour. It isn't acceptance, gratefulness or welcoming. There hasn't been enough time yet to consider the detailed impact of the tumour, nor of my shortened life expectancy. But I feel a gradual awe-filled scientific understanding of what is happening to me. A sense of wonder and amazement that I've not felt since my biology classes at school. It's like when I first began to understand osmosis and then genetics, and how they were both primary foundations for every living thing. This is *life* happening. It's nature doing what nature does. Never so much have I felt my life to be both irredeemably small and insignificant, yet at the same time so individual and important. The strangest contradiction: a death sentence making me feel so alive.

Though it's a 100-mile round trip to Cambridge, I decide to cycle to the appointment. It feels like a little insult to the tumour, but also a physical expression of the body that I am. The cells, and muscles and bones, the osmosis and genetics that are still working. And working fine.

The brain surgeon doesn't comment on my cycling shorts and shoes as I clip-clop into his office. He takes my scans, and like the two surgeons before him repeats the vital information. Large tumour. Probably a low-grade glioma. Stable-looking, but ultimately incurable. I can't help but ask for more. I ask him what it looks like: death from a brain tumour.

"It's a long, long time until we have to consider that," he says.

"Yes, but what can I expect?"

"Well, there will be radiotherapy and chemotherapy." Yes, I know this. I mean after the radiotherapy. After the chemo. When the tumour is back.

"There is likely to be little pain," the doctor's nurse says, finally getting what I'm asking. "In most cases, people – you – will sleep more and more, and then people just don't wake up again."

A peaceful passing into the night. Was this what I'd wanted to hear? Did I instead want thrashing and pain; crawling into a ball on my hospital bed; ripping IV drips from my arms; speaking through a gas mask in a croaky voice, asking my wife to finally let me go?

I cycle the 50 miles back from Cambridge, but this time the journey is melancholy. I realise the last couple of weeks have not been me gently coming to terms with my illness. It has been neither a philosophical adventure nor an abnormally quick understanding and stoic acceptance of my tumour. It has been the opposite.

I have been in shock. Perhaps I still am. I've been putting on a fake face, almost showing off because *something was happening*. I'm the centre of attention. I've been wearing a plaster cast on my arm and doing the rounds – parents, doctors, consultants, nurses – asking them to sign it to show how calm and rational I'm being. Over that 50-mile return journey the truth sets in. There is nothing exciting or thrilling here. Just a dying 35-year-old man. Soon, perhaps as soon as at the end of this cycle ride, I need to accept what has happened for what it really is. And think deeply about the consequences.

About two-thirds of the way into the cycle home, I have a deep epileptic seizure. The first since my daughter's birthday. The first since the doctor walked up the drive a month ago. I have to leap off the bike and stand holding myself up against a hedge. I'm on a blind corner on a tight country road. I can see neither from where I've come nor to where I'm heading.

Searching for a 'yes'

I HAVE ON a piece of paper a list, a dozen or so friends and family who I know I have to call and tell them I have a brain tumour. Sarah and I sat on the sofa the night before and drew up the list as if we were planning next year's Christmas cards. Like with my parents, I know it's me that needs to break the news. Sarah will have her own friends to tell.

I have to *call* my friends, that's the worst of it. I have always hated the phone. It's the small talk that precedes every conversation, the difficult and stilted chat if there's noise in the background, the never quite knowing if the person you're speaking to is doing what you probably are doing too – trying to talk to them, but also doing something else: tidying up, cooking the tea, checking emails. I like to look people in the eye, particularly when there's news to share, whether good or bad. It's the reason that I never pick up. I need to know a call is coming, to plan ahead for it. For the phone, I need space.

I take my list into the bedroom. For a quarter of an hour I stare at the handset like a teenager plucking up the courage to ask someone in their class for a date. What if they're not in? Leave a message? What if they're in, but there's a baby or a visitor or a favourite TV programme in the background? This will be hard enough, without having to feel I'm interrupting.

I have the calls planned: the buildup, the punchline, the slow release of the details. For the rest, I can answer I don't know, that we're trying to find out, but mostly that we're just waiting. I dial the first number and my good friend Dan picks up within a couple of rings.

I don't remember the exact conversations I have that day, but they all go something like this. I move on from introductions and small talk within a matter of seconds. I don't want to get caught up because otherwise my news will seem inappropriate or even more uncomfortable to share.

I'm calling with some bad news, actually. I've been having some tests and I have a brain tumour. It's not good news, I'm afraid. No, they say surgery isn't an option. I was having epileptic seizures on the bike. We're pretty shook up right now. We've known for a week or so, just coming to terms. Trying to understand what's going on. There are lots of questions, we just have to wait.

As I relay the information, I'm walking up and down the cracks in our wooden flooring, pointing my toes at knots in the wood. Turning then walking back up the plank, trying to balance. Watching my feet, just like my family doctor had done when he'd first told me.

And then I feel it. It's the first time I can pin down the emotion though it's something I've been feeling since day one. I feel guilt. I feel guilt that I've introduced something unwanted and unclean into other people's lives. The brain tumour has happened to me, but I'm the bearer of bad news that will affect them. I've ruined their night, perhaps their week, perhaps much longer than that.

I find myself saying sorry, *I hate to tell you like this, I feel bad.* I ask them how they are. If they are alright. I think of my family doctor and how long and lonely that walk up the drive to my house must have been. It's all so crushingly sad, I can't help but well up. At the other end of the line I hear broken voices too. I don't expect a response. I don't know what I would say in their position.

They ask the right questions: not so much about the detail of my illness, but about me and Sarah and Erin and Reid.

How are we? Am I healthy now? What further tests do I need to have? How can they help: babysitting, a visit, or – most touchingly and generous of all – would I like them to call people and tell them the news for me?

No one asks how long I've got, or tells me about other brain tumour patients they know. The conversation is about right now, not about the future. I feel warmth and I feel love. But when I put the phone down, I stare blankly at the next name on the list and my heart starts beating quickly and my mouth goes dry again. It's back to the start. The next call isn't going to be any easier to make than the last one.

I am a coward. I make four phone calls and afterwards I can make no more. I am in bits. I lie on the bed and crush the list in my hand. I lie there staring at the wall, knowing that the last call I made – the fourth – was the last call I will ever make to break the news. I hate myself for it, but I know that tomorrow, perhaps the day after, I will write an email and send it to the rest. Impersonal, unkind, cowardly. But I hope the recipients will understand.

But there are two people – a couple who are very good friends – I know I have to tell personally. It can't be a phone call. They are on holiday together, not far from where I live. My text invites them to drop in on their way home tomorrow. A bite to eat and a quick catch-up to break up their homeward journey? I desperately want them to say 'yes'. I desperately want them to say 'no'.

They arrive and it is with the usual glee that we greet each other. They swing the children around, and we all pat their dog. Sarah goes off to make coffee, and they come into the living room and ask what's the latest?

I tell them.

She begins to cry. They both rise from their places and instinctively embrace me. We hang there for seconds, just feeling each other's warmth. Sarah returns with the coffee and the conversation starts. This is a couple who like detail. He would start taking notes if he had his laptop to hand. We try to ask them about their holiday, but first there are queries to answer, clarifications to offer. They ask sensible and sensitive questions, and I note them myself as things to put in my coward's email when I send it out tomorrow.

And then we talk about brain tumours no more. We talk about holidays and cycling and children and mutual friends. And then they suggest we make plans to take a holiday together in the summer.

The summer.

The future. My friends have opened up, absorbed my information, and now are already talking about our future together. I feel in love with them, overjoyed, positive and uplifted. For me, the future had been all about the second MRI due in three months' time. The most important medical test of my life. Now we have a holiday, and it'll be during the week between the MRI and the results day. We'll spend the week walking and cycling, eating pub lunches and playing board games together. It is the very best idea.

We share lunch, then hug some more and then they leave. The positivity they brought with them hangs in the air but not for long enough. Soon, the house is quiet again. Just me, Sarah and the children. We speak of darker thoughts; despair replaces the hopefulness we've just shared. Sarah tells me she's realised she'd never used the word 'devastated' accurately before. Now she knows what it really means.

Though we're together to support each other, it's hard when you're both equally low. Before this, we might take it in turns to haul each other from whatever shallow pit one or the other might occasionally fall into. Now we're both down and there's no one to pull us out. There's solace in the children, blissfully unaware as kids are, and that's something to cling to. But otherwise the house echoes with everything we now know and there's nothing to fill up the gaps. To absorb the sadness bouncing off every wall. The prospect of a weekend like this is almost oppressive, but we don't know what else to do.

The phone rings and I notice it's Dan, the first person I'd called the day before. Probably just checking I'm alright. "What are you doing tomorrow," he says, the tone of his voice bouncing with excitement. I almost say 'oh, you know, dying from a brain tumour'. I know he would have laughed, but the way I was feeling I'm not sure it would have been a joke.

"Nothing much."

"Perfect," he says. "Because we're coming to see you."

What I have, I tell people in the email, is what doctors suspect is a low-grade glioma brain tumour. I write it as a Q&A, based on the questions I'd been asked by other friends when I'd told them over the last couple of days.

These are tumours that grow from the fatty glial cells that, amongst other things, act like a lubricant in the brain, stopping the white and grey matter from rubbing up against each other as we go about our daily business. Not very glamorous.

My brain tumour, at that time, is approximately five centimetres by four centimetres, another four centimetres deep. That's pretty big for a brain tumour, and because it pushes up against parts of my brain responsible for my right-hand side and my speech, it causes mild seizures, called partial or focal fits. Although I've only ever had these seizures while riding my bike – and no one is quite sure why that would be – it means I cannot drive and I may never drive again.

Thankfully, I write, mine is probably a grade II tumour which makes it low grade. The scale is I to IV. Grades III and IV are full-on brain cancer and not very good news. For the time being my tumour is most likely to be stable though it cannot be operated on. But at some time in the future, it will transform into a higher grade. There's also the potential for it to continue growing in my skull, pushing further on my brain and gradually impairing my functions that way.

I write that doctors can't give me an accurate prognosis. Every tumour is different, every patient is different. I will have a biopsy some time, but not now. Even then, there's only so much we're ever going to know. There's bound to be more information to come over the next weeks and months, even years.

It feels like we've come a long way in recent weeks, but when I look at it distilled in an email it doesn't seem like much at all. I read it again and can't but add a selfish note. I don't really feel up to talking too much about it on the phone right now. But if you want to get in touch, a short note to let us know you're thinking about us would be very welcome.

Friends say it was very like me to write a briefing about my tumour, and showed how I tend to approach most things. Methodical, thinking about what people might want to know. Detailed and rational, honest and realistic.

I consider it a compliment.

How many brain surgeons do you have to consult to believe and trust what they're saying? For me, three was more than enough.

The first said he was sorry but, because my tumour was wrapped around parts of my brain vital for movement and speech, it could not be removed. He also said it was natural to want to seek a second opinion.

So I went for a private consultation with one of the top brain tumour surgeons in the UK. Within 60 seconds of seeing my MRI scans, he concurred with my first surgeon's opinion. Removal was not something he would attempt. Doing so would be folly.

I'd heard what I needed to hear, but I ended up with a

third opinion anyway. This surgeon was highly respected, a patron of the British-based Brain Tumour Charity. His professional and medical opinion was exactly the same as the first two. Mine was not a tumour that could be operated on without doing more damage.

What does a rational person do in this situation? Three expert brain surgeons all concurred exactly with each other. It was the end of the matter. Removal of the tumour was not an option.

But some friends, family and others were not so sure. They suggested I keep looking for a surgeon who *would* take out the tumour. One was suggested who was based in Dublin, Ireland. Apparently he'd operated on someone at work's husband. Another's suggested surgeon was in Canada. He was less cautious than English surgeons with what he'd attempt, I was told. Another suggestion was to track down some wondrous brain tumour surgeon in Germany.

All three would cost lots of money to see. Then more money to have the surgery done. But a 'yes' would be a 'yes'. Surely that's better than a 'no'? I read these emails and heard these suggestions with interest, but how could I take them seriously? Was I supposed to roam the world until I found a doctor that would tell me what I wanted to hear? It is the understandable journey some cancer patients attempt to make. But its pursuit is deeply flawed. One that leads to patients spending huge sums of money and investing huge amounts of hope and emotional turmoil.

If I had gone to see the surgeon in Dublin and he'd met me face to face and seen my scans, and then he'd told me that indeed my other doctors were right, that my tumour wasn't removable, what should I do next? Go to Canada?

What if the Canadian surgeon said 'no' too? Do I then go to Germany?

What if the German doctor then said 'yes'? I'd have seen

five surgeons who'd said 'no', that it would be too dangerous. But finally, at my sixth attempt, I'd have found one who would do it. Hooray. Pull out the drill and scalpels, this German doctor is about to save my life.

Really? What happened to the credibility of the five previous doctors? They were credible enough when I decided to go and see them. Should I now trust their opinions less because they said 'no' while the sixth surgeon says 'yes'? Has he suddenly become super-credible because he assents when five of his colleagues refused? Of course not. In fact, the opposite should be true. A doctor who says he'll operate when five medical colleagues, with equal or even more experience in brain tumours, have said 'no' should surely make me very suspicious. I should trust him *less* than the other five. To go under the German surgeon's knife would be irrational in the extreme, even if that's what I might desperately want. Of course, there's a chance that the German would succeed and the other five were wrong. But given what the other five have said, would I be willing to find out?

Or what if, by chance, I'd gone and seen the German first? Should I then still go to see the Irish and Canadian surgeons anyway, to get their recommendations? Or does my search stop in Germany? If I'd heard the same conclusions in a different order, would this lead to a different final decision?

For me this was an easy decision to make. I wasn't about to chase around the world looking for a green light when all the others lights were red. But unfortunately, even in the extreme case of brain tumours and deadly cancers, patients and their families play exactly this game. They search out that elusive 'yes' when everyone else has said 'no'. It usually costs them an enormous amount of money, and the outcomes are often the same as they would have been. More often, they are worse than if they'd taken their doctors' advice.

You have to try anything

I'M SPEAKING AT a conference on charity marketing. It's my own event and one of the highlights of my working year. I'm standing at the front, one of the star turns. Sixty charity marketing professionals are looking up at me, some with expectant pens poised at their notebooks. I'm standing there and I'm talking, going through my presentation as planned. Bringing points to a crescendo, watching lights switch on in the eyes of some of my audience members as they realise how this idea or that might be turned to advantage in their own organisations. I'm cracking a few jokes and they're laughing in the right places. In a moment, we'll break for coffee. Some will come to the front to clarify points, some clutching their own marketing asking me to take a quick glance over it. We'll talk, network, laugh a little.

I'm on the stage and I'm talking and I'm smiling. But I'm not there. Inside, I feel nothing. I'm going through the motions. An automaton. The words leave my mouth and my body is working, but my mind is dulled. I hear my voice in my head, distinct from the words coming from my mouth. And what I hear is: *you don't know. When I invited you here, when you paid your event fee, I was a different person. Now I'm standing in front of you and I'm not the same. You don't know that your speaker's life has changed forever.*

A thin sheet is draped over those first weeks after diagnosis. We must have got up in the mornings, we must have gone to work, and spent time with the children. We cooked meals and attended birthday parties, called up friends and made visits. I must have met clients, spoken at conferences. But I couldn't have been there, could I? Not really there. I look out at my conference audience and I'm nearing the end of my session. On the outside I'm building my final points, offering final tips, some messages to take home. Inside, I'm hearing: *I don't want to do this anymore. That's enough.*

It's not just the job, it's everything. I just want to go home. I want to close the blue gate at the end of our driveway. I want to gather my wife and children together and lie down with them on our big bed and hold them close to me and just go to sleep. To hide away until all this has passed.

"Life goes on," I say to people who ask how I'm doing. "You can't live in panic every moment," my wife says too. But inside, we are crumbling. We know a little about the future, but not enough to grasp. Only chances and possibilities, an endless list of maybes. When I have to book an appointment, my first thought is whether I will even still be alive.

The conference is the end of the line, my last real commitment on the near horizon. There are a few last writing projects for clients but mostly my diary is clear. The remainder of the spring and then the summer spreads out in front of me like an unanswered question. We decide to go away. I love Spain and this, I think, could be my last chance. My last holiday with my wife and kids. My last chance to see them swim in the sea or dig their toes into the sand to escape the heat of the scorching grains on top. My last chance to watch them eat ice-cream, or to watch as they laugh and make fun as I squirm at the idea of eating mussels and snails. I want to drink every drop of each of them.

I look back on these thoughts now and I'm embarrassed. In those first months, I'd been given no indication my life was even close to being in immediate danger. I'd been told to go away for three months. An MRI in the summer would tell us more and then we'd prepare a plan for what comes next. Every scientific paper I read told me more about my brain tumour and mostly what I learned was good news. But even with this knowledge, every moment I lived felt urgent. Every graph has outliers. Half of people with low-grade gliomas will be dead in five or six years, but *this* person with *this* low-grade glioma could easily be dead long before that.

If the second MRI is bad news, then maybe I'll have to go into treatment right away. Radiotherapy and chemotherapy. The slow ebbing would begin. My last chances would have already been spent. The epilepsy drugs make my mind thick with fugg, I'm too sleepy to think straight. My wife and I feel desperate and impulsive. We should live our lives in Technicolor, we say, because who knows what tomorrow will bring? We definitely have three months left, but theoretically that could be all. So do we sit at home with the gate closed and the covers pulled up? Or do we bet our lives on the worst and live the next few weeks like they are the last?

The trip away offered an understanding of how I'd already become something new. I'd given up my pass to what Susan Sontag called the 'kingdom of the well' and had replaced it with the 'kingdom of the dying.' I have to pay more for travel insurance because, for the first time, I have to tick a box labelled 'any other ongoing medical conditions'. It's annoying, but again brings with it a strange satisfaction of belonging to my new tribe. A badge to wear. I sport an armband, a chain and dog tag around my neck about my epilepsy.

We choose a small, comfortable cottage on the south coast of Spain, near Chiclana de la Frontera. It is a private place, with twin beds for the children, our own kitchen and the sun streaming through the patio doors each morning. The children are wide-eyed when we arrive, running around our holiday home opening cupboards, jumping on beds, trying to work the TV. And then we take them outside, and they see the swimming pool – our own private swimming pool, our life in Technicolor – and we're quickly tearing into our luggage to get their costumes and they're begging us to blow up their armbands. Soon we will go to a busy Spanish market, or walk along the seafront, or eat tapas in an empty restaurant. Then we'll be back at the holiday home and back in the swimming pool until way past their bedtime. Making a simple salad and slicing Spanish cheese, a cold beer from the fridge. It all takes on extra meaning.

One windy day, we go down to the beach and the waves rise up so high it is unsafe for the children to swim. They play in the sand as I head out alone, swimming out of my depth and allowing myself to be thrashed around by the force of the sea. My head rattles around on my shoulders. I feel myself gasping for breath, swallowing water as I open my mouth to find some air. The very highest waves push me to the bottom and onto the sand below. They powerfully cascade into me time and again, offering me little break between. When I emerge from the water and walk back down the beach I notice the dog-tag from around my neck has been torn away.

Later in the week when the sun is going down and the children are in bed, I sit with my feet dangling into the water thinking of the days gone by and watching each star as it gradually unfolds itself out of the dimming sky. I'm happy. Genuinely delighted with my life. You can take me down now, I think. Take me down because whatever my brain tumour does to me I will always have had right now.

Not every moment of the holiday is worry-free. Every afternoon has brought its usual irresistible need to sleep. (At least in Spain, with its culture of siestas, I am in good company.) Despite my happiness and comfort, I am oversensitive and irritable. My wife finds driving stressful, and

I find it just as stressful to sit only on the passenger side. One day we visit a fiesta, packed with fairground rides, horse displays and balloon sellers. The noise from the rides and the crowds, the insistent and whiny pleas from my children for treats feel unbearable. They ring in my ears so loud and oppressive that I have to leave the fair. Even our Technicolor holiday has its limits.

The holiday was a time to take stock. To spend car journeys, the children exhausted and asleep in the back, talking about the future near and far. We spoke of my new detachment when I was speaking at conferences and my ambivalence even as I worked on the few remaining writing projects I had. Sarah spoke of her need to be with me and to be with the family. Our busy life, sometimes passing like ships in the night, exchanging childcare like a relay baton, was something we once thrived upon. Now it was something that no longer fitted. How much time together had we already missed?

By the time we boarded our plane at Seville, I had decided not to continue working as a charity copywriter and consultant for the time being. I couldn't be authentic, I couldn't offer my whole self to those who deserved the best of me. What I was going to do instead, I hadn't yet decided. I wasn't sure I was going to do anything at all for a while. At the end of the summer, my four-year-old daughter would be starting school. This could be my last opportunity to be with my children fully, to offer them the deepest attention I now found so difficult to offer my work. After that, my children's own obligations to their education and to their own life journeys would begin.

I still had my second MRI scan on the immediate horizon, but even if the result was stability in my brain tumour, I decided I would take the remainder of the summer off. To go cycling and enjoy the sunshine. To go on day trips, and cook with the children, to play with them and share picnics under our plum tree.

I would also take time to research and understand my condition in even more detail. To ask every question, perhaps to develop my own opinion. And I would share what I learned along the way: about cancer, about cycling, about myself, about life and about death. I've been a writer since I was a teenager. For 24 years, I have worked as a professional wordsmith. Now I would do what writers do when they get a brain tumour. I would write about it.

A TV documentary about the miracle brain cancer doctor, Dr Stanislaw Burzynski. He is the world's most controversial figure in oncology. For 40 years he has been selling a potential treatment for cancer, but the American authorities only allow him to do it because he's doing so as a clinical trial. Critics say that Dr Burzynski has never published solid evidence that his antineoplaston therapy works, and some argue it does far more harm than good. Children, claims the Texas Children's Hospital close to his treatment centre, frequently end up there with their health in a perilous state thanks to his treatment.

"He must believe in what he's doing, but I have not been convinced by the existing scientific literature that his therapy has any efficacy," Dr Jeanine Graf, medical director of the paediatric intensive care unit at the Texas Children's Hospital told a BBC documentary. "I would not seek out care from him for any of my loved ones nor would I recommend it for any of my patients."

Other critics says that his success is no better or worse than conventional cancer treatment would be. Though it is certainly far more expensive.

Still, families from all over the world head to his Texas lab. They pay many tens of thousands of pounds for a treatment that has never been proven to work, and for decades has been no more than a clinical trial. Dr Burzynski offers a 'yes', or at least an 'it might work', when traditional medicine has said nothing more can be done.

"The NHS are telling me my daughter is going to die. This man is telling me he can cure her," says Lucy Petagine, mother of 18-month-old Luna from the UK. The parents took Luna to see Dr Burzynski after three conventional operations on her brain tumour failed to make her better.

Nobody knows how Dr Burzynski's treatment is even supposed to work. His results are not published in any form that is accepted by the scientific community, a position other oncologists say is unethical. Luna's own doctors advised the family not to go to Texas, telling them they would not know how to treat her when she came back. But like hundreds of families every year, Luna's family were desperate. Desperate enough to go with the one doctor that gave them a 'yes', the one doctor who – unlike every other expert – said he could keep her alive.

Dr Burzynski's treatment didn't work for Luna.

Lucy Petagine told the BBC documentary, "I think it gave us another year. If I hadn't have gone I would be sat here without my daughter saying I wish I'd tried it. And you can't put a price on hope … at the end of the day, as a parent with a child that was dying, and you're told this child's going to die, you would try anything. Anything."

Why do we believe in this magic formula to 'try anything' when it comes to cancer? It rolls so easily off the tongue in response to the disease, particularly when you're trying to console someone or fear you are going to lose a child: well, you've just got to try anything, haven't you?

But have you? Do you really have to 'try anything', even if there is no evidence that the *anything* works? Even if there is contradictory evidence? Even if it has been shown *not* to work?

There's a difference between 'there's no evidence that it does not work' and 'there's no evidence that it does'. The second assumes that tests have been made, that the proposed cure or action has received some scientific analysis, and that proposed cure has been found wanting. There is good reason for believing it does not cure cancer.

The first – there's no evidence that it does not work – sounds like the foundation to pursue a proposed cure. But really it shows the irrationality of the 'try anything' mistake. There are many millions of things that have not been proven to *not* cure cancer, but mostly because many millions of things have never been tried. That does not mean they are a potential cure, nor that they are sensible to pursue.

In the 'try anything' world, who gets to decide what the *anythings* we should try are? Is there a lowest bar above which *anything* must rise to be justified as worthy of pursuit? Or do we really mean *anything* – whatever someone proposes because, well, you never know?

What if I proposed that blowing up 100 red balloons could cure your cancer? I suspect it's never been tested though I also suspect oncologists would strongly suggest it won't work. But it might! Indeed, blowing up 100 red balloons has never been disproven: there's no evidence that it *does not* work. Therefore, I should try it, shouldn't I?

I am being cynical. Of course, blowing up 100 red balloons will not cure cancer. How ridiculous. But why is that any more ridiculous than many of the other *anythings* we should try? What if I put my *anything* into a pill or a bottle, is that preferable? More legitimate? What if I pump my *anything* into your arm? What if I give it a scientific-sounding name? Is it now less ridiculous than the balloons? Does that *anything* now become the type of *anything* we should try?

What if I told you to meditate? To eat garlic supplements? To have colonic irrigation with coffee enemas? To get or change your religion? To think positively? Are they more, or less, ridiculous *anythings*? Are all *anythings* equal, or are some *anythings* more worthy than others?

If there is a line between the *anythings* we should try and *anythings* we shouldn't, and if there is a line between a ridiculous *anything* and a non-ridiculous *anything*, then who gets to draw the line? Who gets to decide?

Among alternative medicine practitioners, for example, there is nowhere near agreement about what is ridiculous and what is legitimate as treatment when it comes to cancer. Some think another's cure or treatment is bogus. In turn, others say the same about theirs. It's not good enough for this line to be blurred. In the world of treatments and cures, it's not enough to urge people to try things and just see how they get on.

There is something that does draw a clearer line for us. It is called scientific research. And it derives its authority from clear rules for scientific testing. There is a way to draw the line as neatly as possible. That is the way to see which side of the line any proposed *anything* sits. Has the proposed cure or prevention been proven to work? Is it biologically plausible? Has it been tested in animals? Is it backed by the majority of the scientific establishment?

If not, then shouldn't it sit on the ridiculous side – along with the 100 red balloons – until it has earned the right to cross? That it has 'not been proven *not* to cure cancer' is, like so much in this disease, merely playing with words. A semantic somersault that gets us nowhere nearer to the truth.

But what am I supposed to do? Obediently heed my doctors' advice? When they have run out of options, should I sit here and wait to die? Surely doing something is better than nothing? Something gives me solidity. Something gives my family a focus, something to campaign about, to rally around, to hope for. Something is at least *something*.

Something does give cancer patients and their families a focus, even if that something contains no truth. It is natural to rally around the things we have in common to find direction in our lives. I question not the understandable act of rallying or even the act of searching or wanting something to cling to. But I challenge the hole into which it is too easy to fall: that the *something* around which we rally in times of crises becomes legitimatised only by the act of the rallying itself. Rallying is understandable and natural, but that doesn't make the *something* any more credible.

I want to utter the unutterable. I want to tell parents who go off in pursuit of a promised miracle cure for their child's cancer that they are wrong. They are deluded, blinded by grief, distracted. I'd like to say to those who work towards or donate to such rallying calls that they are mistaken, however united in doing at least *something* it makes them feel. I want to say that everyone should ask more questions. Be more doubtful. Think twice, three times. I want to say that so much more time could have been shared as a family together, understanding and loving, making the most of what is left, instead of chasing the end of a rainbow. That that time and effort could have been spent raising money for cancer charities.

But I can't say these things. The family is not wrong in these terrible circumstances. It is easy to criticise from my armchair when others are so close to the barricades. I can't judge whether it is wrong or right to choose *something*, even when that *something* is most often nothing. There is no blame to be laid at the cancer patient's door, at those of the family and friends, the donors and those who answer the rallying call. We see pain and we want to try to ease it. We have done it before and we will do it again.

However, in some cases there are those who benefit from our need to 'try anything'. There are those who are mistaken, those who are deluded, those who are irrational and those who are all three. There are those who tell us they have the secret to solving the cancer riddle with non-conventional treatments.

I cannot blame the families who grieve, the patients who are dying, those who when when stripped of everything else will look to any *anything* that is offered. I cannot blame the supporters and donors who are guilty of nothing but their own benevolent humanity.

But those who offer us that *anything* without a fair, accurate and accountable foundation benefit from our hope and desperation. The vulnerability of cancer patients and those who love them gives enormous power to those who would offer a cure or treatment. Those with such power should be held accountable for how they earn it and how they wield it.

We do not have the right to assume that power by writing the word "cancer expert" in a book or on a website. It should not be conjured out of the air or bought over the internet. That power and responsibility should only be earned by results, proof and accountability.

For every dollar or pound paid for a treatment that is without sound proof, a dollar or pound is lost to genuine research and scientific testing. A dollar or pound is lost to medical research that *has* earned the responsibility it claims, and that is held accountable for the power it wields. Mainstream medicine has to justify its claims. It is held responsible for its successes and failures.

When a cancer patient instead allows those who cannot be held accountable to treat them, mainstream doctors and oncologists are often deprived of the opportunity to make someone better; or at least to learn more about what they cannot achieve and why they cannot achieve it.

Those pursuing unproven alternative medicine often cannot participate in medical trials. Mainstream doctors may not even know their patients are also pursuing alternative treatments. Their data and experience, information about their conditions and treatments, may not be able to contribute to our wider knowledge about cancer. Knowledge that leads to slow step-by-step improvements and medical discovery that benefits everyone. Their data is invisible to those with the tools and expertise to use it in their genuine evidence-based (and accountable) search for a cancer mitigation or cure.

How much slower is genuine cancer research moving because of the unearned assumption of power by those who take the patients and the money that conventional scientific research so desperately needs?

It is late July. I know the drill this time because I learned it three months ago. I don't have to ask directions to the Colchester MRI department. I already know that this time I'll be scanned on the inside machine, not in the mobile version still sitting out in the car park. It's been three months since I stepped into that lorry as a man full of health and then stepped out with a brain tumour.

There's nothing to be afraid of today. It's just pictures. This is the most important medical test I've had in my life, but it'll be 10 days before I have to return to the hospital to be told the results. Today is just about whizzing and buzzing, another cannula into my arm, a cold blood-dye visible to the MRI going into my veins, up my shoulder, through my heart and into my central nervous system.

There's about 45 minutes of MRI scanning, but I'm numb to it. It's just something I have to do. I feel emotionless as I lie there, more concerned about staying absolutely still than what the images will reveal. It feels routine and I've prepared. Tracksuit bottoms, no metal on my clothing, my keys safely stored away. There are still no metal shards in my eyes. When it's finished, I thank the radiographer. No doctor comes to look at my scans. They remove the cannula and I'm free to go. I cycle home. The imaging is done.

In the afternoon we go on holiday again. It's the week

away with our good friends whose immediate response to my news was to say, "Let's go away together". They have their own medical issue to deal with: IVF treatment with their own watch-and-wait now to see if an embedded fertilised egg will hold. For all of us, a holiday will take our minds away from doctors' offices and images for a short time at least. We head towards Chichester, close to the south coast of England. Another private cottage, similar to ones we've hired together a number of times before. There are plans to share time walking, sightseeing, cycling, and laughing and drinking late into the night. The company is, as always, good. But the weather is terrible. It's hard to enjoy a long walk in the pouring rain, and the bike I've brought with me goes almost untouched for the duration. The beach is cold and windy and drenched.

My fragile friend needs to rest. She doesn't want to go far from our holiday home, even far from the sofa. I'm feeling low, stressed and tired. I take to bed each afternoon to sleep, and even when I'm awake my sadness is scattered over everything we do. My wife and friend do their best to entertain the children, to make the best of it. Mostly they play games or do local walks while my friend and I sit in the living room together and watch the swimming at the Olympics on TV.

On one rare sunny but windy day, my wife and I muster the strength to head to the beach to allow the kids to at least play in the sand. I join the day trip, but I'm too melancholy to play. Despite the weather improving, the black clouds looming over me are the worst they've been so far. I wrap myself in my coat against the wind and watch my family from a distance, wondering why we're here. I'm so tired I consider lying down there on a damp dune, willing the sand to cover me. I feel vacant and distant. Travel sick in my own body. We want to eat, but there's only a crappy cafe serving limp sandwiches or ice creams that far from match the weather. Sarah offers her usual patience with me, but I can tell the elastic is taut. The worst thing about holidays is that you have to take yourself.

And I feel helpless. I'm no assistance. I want to rise from my tucked-up ball, but my body wants to stay where it is. We snipe on the beach, then argue in the car park. New rain clouds edge over the beach and it starts to pour, first spitting then more determined. "Is this it?" I say to her from beneath my hood. "Am I dying? Is this what dying is? I don't feel very alive anymore. I don't even remember what being alive feels like."

We sit in the car; I lean my head against the window and we hope the weather will clear. We go in search of somewhere to eat, bickering about whether that pub or this would have child-friendly food, or would even be serving food at this time. After too long we find a garden centre with an informal restaurant. There's a kids menu and warming soup. The weather begins to lift and my mood with it. As the children play with crayons and colouring books, I take my wife's hand and apologise. It sometimes feels like I can't carry this. I tell her I know how hard this is on her too, but I feel locked away as if behind inches of glass. I'll break through. I just need to sleep. Tomorrow will be better. I know that while I wait to emerge, she'll be there with the kids trying to be normal. Trying to hide her own distress, so as not to add to mine.

"Don't worry," she says. "No emotion is the final one." It's what she says. It's a quote from Jeanette Winterson's book *Oranges Are Not The Only Fruit*. She's used it with me each time I've felt down, or useless, or frustrated, from long before my diagnosis. I smile and look into her eyes. I look deep and I can see inside there's panic and sadness there, behind the mask she's wearing for me and the children. I love her but don't have the words to express how much. I can say it, but it's not enough. The most I can do is to take back some of the burden from her, but I'm already full. Barely keeping it together. Not keeping it together at all. This is what waiting for results feels like. It is unbearable, yet there is nothing else we can do.

Something we often hear about cancer patients when they've died is that they never complained at all, they took it all with a happy face. But I'm not like that at all. I complain all the time about my health, the unlucky cards we've been dealt. But it is upon Sarah that the burden his piled highest. And I don't have the strength to offer the support for her. Before the day is out, I decide to seek professional help. I will start seeing a counsellor within a few weeks. It's the least I can offer my wife to try to get my head a little more together.

When we arrive back at the house, our friends have had a better day. They are full of smiles and we talk of getting a takeaway meal. I sleep and then we play with the kids. We enjoy each other's company and the pressure is released. We drink a glass or two of wine, a beer and then a whisky, sitting up later than we should. I worry whether the alcohol is clashing with my drugs, making my lowness even lower. The leaflet says to avoid drinking. Maybe stopping alcohol altogether is another thing I can do to chase the black dogs away.

But after such a low day, it's a good night. By the end, we all know the holiday has not run as smoothly as it could have. But it's also been better than us all sitting in our own homes worrying about the future, holding our breath for the next step.

Success and failure

A DAY AFTER we return from our Chichester holiday in early August, I'm due back at the hospital for my results. This is the big one, the first opportunity to assess whether my brain tumour has grown, changed or even turned malignant. I'd met my local oncologist a week before my MRI scan. He is friendly and upbeat, wearing a Wallace & Gromit tie and joking with us about my obsession with cycling. I like him. He talks about my tumour in a blasé way, throwing around five, 10 and 15 years like they're colour handkerchiefs he's pulling out of a hat. If anyone has to deliver my bad news, I'm glad it's him.

Colchester County Hospital is a decrepit, dismal affair of faded yellow corridors. In the blank waiting room, volunteers sell plastic cups of instant coffee and limp cling film-wrapped ham sandwiches from a sad hatch. The room is crowded with people in various states of illness. There are older people with walking frames and younger ones with crutches. There are young adults with faces burned from radiotherapy, others with clumps of hair missing or wearing the signature headscarf of a cancer patient. This is what oncology looks like, I think. This is what my brother faced every day as he went for daily radiotherapy and chemotherapy. Alone. Without me accompanying him even once.

In the corner there is a small library managed by the charity Macmillan Cancer Support, rows of leaflets and booklets. In a hospital years before, I might have shied away from this section, almost as if by browsing cancer leaflets I was in some way invading someone else's illness. Or worse, that I might somehow absorb cancer myself. But now I'm part of the tribe. These leaflets are for me. I find one on self-employment and another on benefits, then a booklet on telling your children you have cancer. Finally, there's a booklet on brain tumours. This one I carefully arrange on the top of the pile as I walk with them in my hand back to my seat. No need to guess what my cancer is. There's no need to be embarrassed, as I am when I see a man with a huge tumour protruding from his neck. I might look perfectly healthy, but look: the booklet says it all. I'm in an oncology waiting room and, yes, I belong.

My name is called. This time it is a yellow line I follow as it winds its way around the corridors towards my oncologist's office. Only when it reaches his office he's not there. He should be here, waiting for me like last time, ushering me into his room with a smile. Instead, I follow the yellow line to the feet of another doctor. A woman I've never met before. A woman with an emotionless face and an impatient manner.

Is this what it does to you? Is this how you end up looking when the friendly oncologist passes the hopeless cases to you? Is this how you look when you have to deliver the bad news? All stern lips and cold eyes. She invites us in, still not smiling as she introduces herself as an oncologist from the department. She asks me how I am.

How am I? I have a brain tumour. I am a dying man. How do *you* think I am? "Fine," I say. "Pretty good. Just, you know, tired from time to time, but that could be the epilepsy drugs…" She's not listening. And I'm not listening to my words either. I'm thinking she should stop asking me how I am, and start *telling* me how I am. Deliver the news then let me go home to cuddle my kids and then go to bed. But she's in no rush.

She talks about my tumour in words I don't understand,

medical jargon as if she's making a presentation at a conference. There are no scans up on her computer screen. Her tone remains flat and matter of fact. She talks about indolence and vascularity and histology and MRI imaging and who knows what else. I'm following as closely as I can, trying to understand, trying to pick out a word or two that resonates. But I'm too nervous, already concerned that I've missed the vital bit. Then, jumbled up in the words she's saying, I hear the word 'stable'. A minute later she repeats the word. Stable.

I say it in my head and then finally understand. I stop her.

"I'm sorry, did you say stable?"

"Yes," she says, as if that's something I should already know. "Stable. There's no noticeable change in your tumour." Then she goes straight back into medical speak, before rising and moving towards the door. The meeting is over. I'm to make another MRI appointment for six months' time.

"But the seizures," I say. "I'm still having seizures. And I feel so tired all the time..." I'm trying to get out all the questions I'd come in with and all the time her hand is reaching towards the door handle. Her sigh of impatience is audible. She's done her job as far as she is concerned. She's talked at me and out of what she's said I've managed to deduce that my tumour is unchanged. She's delivered, what else did I want?

I want party poppers. Balloons. A shake of the hand. A pat on the back. A congratulations. Or at least a smile.

"Listen," she says. She's actually opened the door now and is walking through it. "You're bound to have side effects, aren't you? You've got a brain tumour." And then she's gone.

It takes 10 seconds for my anger at her rudeness to dissipate. Another 10 for my disappointment at being treated so coldly to pass. And then there's just warmth in my heart. Sarah and I walk back along our yellow line, holding hands in silence.

Stable. Neither of us want to utter the words in case we somehow destroy the magic and make it untrue. It's like when you've been to see an excellent film, and don't want to talk about it on the way out because nothing needs to be said.

When we reach the reception desk, it occurs to me. She said to make an appointment for another MRI in six months. Not three months, but six. It's an indication of just how stable my tumour must be. No growth, no malignancy. Go home and get on with your life. The rest of summer, then autumn and winter. Halloween, Christmas, New Year. After three months of fear and stress, six months is a lifetime.

Behind the hospital where we've parked, finally we can no longer keep quiet about the movie we've just watched. We smile and hug and there are tears in Sarah's eyes. We've come through this, and have been granted a reprieve. I want to text everyone I know, tell them I'm off death row. "The news could not have been better," I say as we get into the car. "Perfect."

It's only later that I allow myself to process how terse the doctor had been. It's something that will always taint what should have been a happy moment of our lives after three months of little but suffering and worry. It takes me months to think it through, to understand just how unkind the doctor had been. There was no malice; there was just a lack of thought. When there's only one thing you need to hear – good or bad – a little sensitive thought goes a long way. I decide I will move my care to London.

What would it take for proponents of non-mainstream medicine to admit that they got it wrong? As a high school philosophy student I learned about the 'procrustean' tendency, the practice of changing the facts or ignoring inconvenient ones that don't fit with your preconceived theory or belief. In alternative cancer treatments the procrustean tendency runs savagely free. Even some of the biggest champions of alternative medicine have blamed other factors for the death of cancer patients rather than admit that the treatment they were pursuing or promoting didn't work.

The British alternative medicine proponent Chris Woollams' daughter Catherine had an aggressive malignant brain tumour. With the help of his diets, supplements, cranial osteopathy, hands-on healing as well as yoga and exercise classes, Woollams claimed that his daughter had, for a time, successfully staved off her cancer. But eventually she died. Doctors, he says, gave Catherine six months. She had survived for three-and-a-half years.

And it is a fact that survival of this length for a grade IV glioma is unusual. But it is far from unheard of. According to the American Brain Tumor Association, one in 10 glioblastoma patients live over five years. Cancer Research UK says around six in 100 grade IV glioma patients survive for five years or more after diagnosis. But an article by Chris Woollams on the website for cancerActive, a charity which he and Catherine helped to establish, at least appears to show a procrustean tendency in his claims.

"Catherine did extremely well for nearly three years. Sadly, flushed with all this success, Catherine returned to the more normal life of a 24-year-old, going back to smoking and drinking, and stopping the exercise and supplements. What does go through the mind of a young woman when told she has 'beaten' the unbeatable? The cancer returned."

Woollams seems to believe that because his daughter's cancer returned, his regime wasn't properly followed. There seemed to be no question that his regime itself might not work. Nor that it might have been merely coincidence that his daughter followed his regime and lived as long as she did. There was no acknowledgement that Catherine could have been an outlier: living for that long was definitely possible within the scope of her diagnosis. For Woollams the regime had to be right, so something else must have been amiss for her eventual death.

In the same way, Jessica Ainscough – an Australian lifestyle and fitness guru – came to acclaim for rejecting conventional medicine for the cancerous sarcoma growing in and on her arm. It's a type of cancer that affects fibrous tissues, as well as bones and nerves. She was widely praised for her brave and anti-establishment stance, and set herself up as 'The Wellness Warrior', launching her own suite of health products and then marketing them (and herself) through TV talk show appearances. Appearances which took her rejection of the mainstream treatment as their key hook.

When it became clear that her daily dose of coffee enemas (called Gerson therapy), an organic diet and meditation was doing nothing to stop the recurrence of her cancer, people posting on her blog continued to praise her position. But they claimed that if she wasn't getting better it must be because she wasn't doing Gerson therapy correctly. They then took the opportunity to recommend their own swathe of alternative methods. Ainscough appears to have had a change of heart about conventional medicine in her final months, but by then it was too late. She died in early 2015.

Procrusteanism is pervasive in alternative cancer prevention and cure. But it does not stand up to logical scrutiny. Philosopher Karl Popper posited an important test for measuring whether there is meaning in scientific and religious claims. He suggested that if a theory is to be taken seriously, those who propose it must be able to define what it would take for that theory to be falsified. If my theory is that 'all swans are white' then I have to admit that if anyone was to find a swan that was black, or pink, or green, then my theory would be proved false. It doesn't matter if no one *does* observe a black swan, it matters that I *know and declare* what it would take for my claim to be wrong.

Apply that logic to alternative medicine and it reveals how meaningless some cancer prevention or cure theories are. What would it have taken, for example, for David Servan-Schreiber to allow that his anticancer theories might be wrong? He died from the cancer that had started the whole exercise in the first place, yet on his deathbed he refused to admit an error in his approach.

Like Servan-Schreiber, in her book *Mum's NOT Having Chemo*, Laura Bond claims we all have the power to beat cancer, or avoid getting it in the first place, by looking at our diet and our mental state: do we have the 'cancer personality'? The basis of her book is that it's just a case of continuing to look until we find the right prevention, therapy or cure for us and our cancer. In the introduction to *Mum's NOT Having Chemo* she writes that the treatments her mum has found most helpful "like infrared saunas and energy medicine, for example – have made it into this book. Other treatments, like laetrile (apricot kernels), haven't make the cut. But that's not to say these protocols aren't right for others dealing with the disease. Every cancer is different, every person is different and every treatment plan will be different. There are many paths to recovery…"

In the concluding chapter she writes, "While I hope this book has brought you important information, nothing compares to the innate intelligence of your own intuition. What resonates with you? How does your body feel when you take a new supplement or try a new therapy? Are these things you can discuss with your physician and if not, what's stopping you from finding a doctor who's on the same page as you? The idea that 'cancer is not a one-size-fits-all disease' cannot be emphasised enough: what works for one person might not work for the next."

There's no possibility of her being wrong. If you're not cured, then you didn't find the right treatment or approach for you. If it does cure you, you hit the jackpot and found it. If your doctor doesn't agree with your methods, the methods aren't wrong, you just need to find another doctor. Bond is in the illogical position of being right in every case. Or, as Karl Popper would have it, her claim that we need to keep looking until we find the right cure is not falsifiable.

If alternative medicine won't submit cures and treatments to conventional medical testing, claiming too often that there's something special or even magical about how they work so they don't fit into such a structured regime as medicine and science, then perhaps they should at least submit to the entirely logical question of falsifiability.

Someone has invented the cancer prevention tincture Potion A. Before they start selling Potion A, they must first describe what it would take to conclude that Potion A doesn't work. If someone taking Potion A gets cancer, would that be the time to admit that Potion A doesn't work? What if 10 people taking Potion A get cancer, would that be sufficient evidence that it doesn't work? What about 100?

What about if the number of people taking Potion A who got cancer was the same as the number who would normally be expected to get cancer if they weren't taking it? Can it still be said to work now? If the profferer of Potion A doesn't admit even in those circumstances that it doesn't work, then there's only one place to go. That Potion A actually makes cancer more likely. And what kind of cancer prevention is that?

Somewhere, the inventors have to define what 'Potion A prevents cancer' means. And define it in specific numbers and within boundaries such as age or lifestyle. Testimonials of people who've taken Potion A and haven't (yet) got cancer are not good enough.

The problem is that those who promote these cancer preventions and cures, and those who take them, often only talk in terms of the success they've had. They don't define what *not working* might look like. Those who take cancer prevention therapies and live to 100 claim it is the therapy that got them there, despite the fact that others reach the same age with no such therapy. Those who take the same therapy but *do* get cancer will often point to bad luck, or not doing the therapy correctly. The last thing they will accept is that the cancer prevention they invested in (financially and emotionally) doesn't work.

Those who take cancer cures and do beat their cancer sometimes swear it was the experimental cure, rather than luck or any conventional treatment they also received. "My doctors aren't convinced – but I believe green tea cured my cancer", reads one UK newspaper headline. In a surprising number of survivor testimonies, the patient took both conventional therapies and alternative medicine, but credits the unproven alternative medicine for their survival rather than the proven treatment.

Those who don't cure their cancer with the alternative treatment either blame some other factor (including the chemo, rather than the cancer) or their final thoughts on their treatment are not recorded. Those who claim to have benefited from cancer prevention and miracle cures are happy to tell their success stories on websites, newspapers and in promotional brochures. The dead don't leave testimonials.

Of course, conventional medicine claims to be able to cure cancer too. And yet cancer patients undergoing conventional treatments die every day. So, surely they're no better than alternative medicine?

But it is not the same. The medical use of chemotherapy, for example, is not predicated on the idea that 'chemotherapy always works', only that it 'often works' and 'it works better than doing nothing'. This has been proven for many cancers, but certainly not all. But vitally, the medical testing protocol for chemotherapy, as for any other mainstream treatment, is based on falsifiability. Researchers know before they even begin what it would take for their assertion 'chemotherapy works' to be falsified: if chemotherapy did not lead to more people being cured of a particular cancer than would have been cured of that same cancer without it, then the statement 'chemotherapy works for this cancer' would be false. And for the relevant cancers they would (and indeed do) stop using chemotherapy.

Sometimes scientific trials don't lead to what the researchers thought they would. Their proponents are sometimes wrong. But that doesn't make the scientific method wrong. And it doesn't mean the results aren't still useful. In fact, the opposite is true. Their results contribute to the canon of scientific literature that will further the development of better cures and preventions for the future. In conventional scientific research, proof that something is false is just as valid and important as proof that something is true.

Personal testimonies are the stock in trade of alternative cancer therapies, preventions and even cures. Whether in text or on videos, the websites for these treatments are full of people claiming they benefited from what is on offer.

Some claim they had cancer but it went away after having the treatment or therapy. Others say they had conventional therapy and non-conventional therapy at the same time, but that they're convinced it was the natural treatment that cured them. Others claim to feel better, or that their tumour has reduced in size, or has stopped growing, or that they're now living cancer-free thanks to the therapy.

Testimonies are a must-have in marketing. They offer social proof. If you see someone like you has bought or tried a therapy and it has succeeded for them, then you're more likely to try it yourself. The more testimonies there are, the stronger the social proof is. It's the reason why we're more likely to buy books with lots of stars and lots of reviews on Amazon, rather than those with no reviews and no stars at all. But there are some considerable logical problems with trusting testimonies as proof of the efficacy (rather than the popularity) of a particular treatment, or relying on them alone when making decisions about our own treatments.

First is the difficult-to-accept fact about cancer: it doesn't matter what *you think* cured you or made you feel better. Opinion doesn't come into it, only the biology and science.

Those who are having both conventional therapy and alternative therapy at the same time and who claim they are sure it was the alternative therapy that was responsible for their recovery are the clearest indication of this. They call themselves living proof that the therapy works, but really they're only proof that they are still alive.

If a person is having chemotherapy and coffee enemas at the same time, it doesn't matter that they think it was enemas that cured their cancer or reduced the size of the tumour. The truth is it is far more likely to have been the chemo. The fact that chemo made them feel ill, whereas the coffee helped them to relax and feel better emotionally, is irrelevant to what *actually* affected the cancer.

Yes, chemotherapy is horrible. It makes patients feel awful and compared with it, almost any more 'natural' treatment is going to make someone *feel* better. But that's the point of chemotherapy. It is killing off cells – cancer cells and others – and during treatment that's going to make patients feel very sick indeed. But after chemotherapy has stopped, slowly patients start to recover. And hopefully, the cancer has reduced or even gone away as a result. Whether the patient drank green tea during chemotherapy or took coffee enemas afterwards doesn't make a difference to whether chemo worked.

And this doesn't just apply when mixing conventional and alternative medicine. It applies when a patient decides to forgo traditional cancer treatment and to only take the alternative route. It may well be that a patient honestly believes that the alternative therapy is responsible for their recovery from cancer or the tumour's regress. And that might well be. But without statistics or proof that exactly correlates the therapy with the cancer, it is a claim without sound basis.

It might have been the alternative therapy. But it could also have been some other factor at play: the cancer was not what oncologists thought it was; the cancer spontaneously regressed (this does happen); there was something else that the patient was doing (alongside therapy) that led to the regression; any number of other reasons. Including pure luck. Each is as likely as the other, and it doesn't matter what the patient *feels* was responsible, only what science can prove. And without evidence, it doesn't give that patient – or proponents of that therapy – the right to promote the therapy as a cure for cancer.

'It worked for me' is no evidence at all. It may well be that the therapy *did* lead to the regression of the cancer, but unless the therapy was undertaken as part of a scientifically controlled experiment, a testimony that it did has no credibility. It doesn't add anything to the canon of oncological literature. That's a real shame, because if there is something out there that is 'natural' and alternative that is truly leading to cancer regression, oncologists sure want to know about it.

But wait. If a therapy or cure has 100 testimonies on its website, or 200 people who claim it has cured them, isn't that evidence in itself? Unfortunately not. It is more social proof, that's for sure: it's more likely to *convince* people that it works. But that's not proof that it actually *does* work.

That's because 200 testimonies saying the treatment worked for them tells us nothing about the total number of people using the treatment. If 1,000 people took the treatment, but it didn't work well enough for 800 people for them to be willing or well enough to leave a testimony, then the 200 testimonies we read present to the reader a skewed 'proof' that it is effective.

For those 200 testimonies to offer any kind of proof, we need to know about the others. From the 200 testimonies alone we don't know: how many people are taking the treatment, how many it has worked for, how many it has not worked for, how many it worked for but who didn't want to leave a testimony, how many it didn't work for who didn't want to leave a testimony, how many were not asked to leave a testimony, and – perhaps most importantly – how many people died before being able to give a testimony. And we need to be able to compare that against the results for people in a similar position who didn't take that treatment.

Two hundred positive testimonies are not compounded evidence. They're simply a group of single testimonies piled on top of each other. Each needs to be taken on its own merits, not as part of a group. We don't even know if one patient who is full of praise for the treatment had the same cancer, the same dose, the same frequency or the same exposure to the treatment as the next testimony on the website. There's no way of comparing them.

The problem is that these endless lists of positive testimonies can actually be dangerous. They can lead to desperate patients *believing* a therapy is effective when actually there's no proof that it is.

And those who follow the unproven treatments because of reading so many glorious testimonies, but the treatment doesn't work for them: surely they can only feel that *they* are the problem, not the treatment. They don't live up to the testimony standard. They're not fighting hard enough. Or maybe they feel they're not doing the treatment properly.

Acres of testimonials have shown the treatment works, so if it is failing then it must be their fault.

Patients apparently have so much to tell the world about the efficacy of their alternative treatments, and the proponents of such treatments are surely keen for more patients to take the treatment. So it is hard to understand what is preventing alternative medicine practitioners from carrying out even the most basic of scientifically grounded, controlled tests among the patients who come through their door.

Instead of listing page after page of untrustworthy testimony, practitioners could publish honest – even independently audited – lists of (anonymised) patients who came to their treatment, their time on the treatment and their dose, and the progress of their disease. This is basic statistical work. If a treatment really does work, providing this very basic data could only do good things for marketing it. Patients could even demand that this approach be taken before they begin the therapy or insist on revealing their full cancer history, particularly what mainstream cancer treatment they have also undergone, when asked to leave a testimony.

Only by comparing data can a true picture be gained about any treatment's efficacy. It's what mainstream medicine does, even on a family doctor's surgery level. If it is possible for a family doctor to record this kind of data, it's certainly possible for an alternative practitioner. The often-repeated claim that there's no money to truly test alternative medicine is a red herring. Any simple to understand book on statistics or medical testing can show even the smallest alternative therapist how to do it. Measurables. Key Performance Indicators. Targets. These are the necessary elements of any successful small business and the internet is full of simple ways to measure and show them.

Rather than proof that alternative therapies work, the personal testimony that claims it does is actually the enemy of proof. First, it offers a skewed view to people with cancer about the efficacy of an alternative treatment, hiding possible failures and weaknesses in the therapy. Secondly, publishing only personal testimonies robs mainstream medicine of statistics and information that would help doctors to better understand the ways everyone (not just those who leave a testimony) reacts to and treats their cancer. This prevents researchers from getting an accurate picture of therapies that work and that don't. That research could truly help cancer patients, as well as practitioners of alternatives therapies.

Imagine if researchers were able to gain an accurate, objective picture of those treated by alternative therapies and their outcomes. They could pursue the most promising therapies as an avenue for research. They could try to discover what it is in the alternative therapies that is responsible for their working. They could further refine and perfect them to help treat more cancer patients. Isn't this exactly what alternative medicine proponents want?

The problem with testimonies is that they are, by the very nature, subjective, fallible, subject to bias. They are exactly the opposite of the objective, free from emotion and free from bias data that is the basis for sound medical evidence. Testimonies are anti-evidence.

Our knee jerk reaction when we see dozens of positive responses to a particular alternative therapy is to be more persuaded that the therapy works. The truth is that 'it worked for me' testimonies thoroughly muddy the waters.

Looks can deceive

WHEN I FIRST revealed my diagnosis to family and friends, I received wave upon wave of support and love. But six months on, I feel I have nothing to show in exchange. I have only a piece of paper carrying the word 'stable', the dismissal to go home and get on with life. I have no surgery scars to brandish, no walking stick to wave. I'm not bedridden or hooked up to a drip. There are no barren patches where my hair has fallen out.

My tumour may be stable, but I do not feel well. It's three months since my second MRI scan and the doctor telling me there's no significant growth in my tumour. I should be larking around, pretending nothing has changed. Getting on with the years of life I've been told will be mine. But I do not feel the health my doctor's conclusion has promised. Neither in my brain nor in my body.

Before the day of diagnosis, I would have one of my mild epileptic seizures perhaps once a month. Since then, the seizures have gradually become more frequent. Where once it might have been about one in ten rides, and only when I was pushing it hard, over more recent times it has become every ride in five, then one in three.

Now I have seizures every time I climb into the saddle, sometimes two or three in a ride, no matter how hard I am working, no matter how fast I turn the pedals. I turn to running instead. But the running soon begins to bring on seizures too. Whichever way I turn the tumour is tracking me, stalking, determined.

The doctor says I am stable, but my epilepsy is telling me something different. If the tumour is not growing, why are the seizures getting more frequent? If the drugs dose I'm gradually increasing aims to dampen down my epilepsy, how can the seizures be consistently getting worse? It's a predictable pattern, week on week. Surely there is something wrong? Growth that the doctor missed. Growth since the last MRI was taken. I have four months left until my next scan, but it doesn't feel like months of freedom. It feels like an unbearable wait.

And it is not just the seizures. In September, I am hit by massive stomach cramps that have me crawling around on the floor for seven hours wondering whether this was just food poisoning or whether my brain has sent satellite cancers around my body and one has lodged in my stomach and was doing what it certainly felt like: eating me up from the inside out.

I manage to wait until 6 a.m. until I finally head to A&E in a taxi, along with a folder of information about my brain tumour. I'm given intravenous pain relief and left to sleep for an hour until a kind hospital doctor tells me I've likely developed a stomach ulcer. If it hasn't been caused by stress, it's certainly not being helped by it. He sends me away with a prescription for high-strength gastric tablets, another daily pill to add to my growing collection.

Most days I wake with a mild headache above my right eye, often with a metallic taste in my mouth. Sometimes there is an electric-like tingling in my jaw, where my broken tooth used to be. There is a bean-shaped lump in my groin, the same size and shape as the one that sat close to my brother's neck and turned out to be lymphatic cancer. I feel slight brain delays, as if my mind is buffering like an internet movie on a bad connection.

I feel like I stumble over my words more often than I used to, and I get them wrong or upside down when I read aloud to my children. And did I always occasionally bump into door frames when I tried to pass through? My chronic tiredness continues, my irritability is more pronounced than ever.

Perhaps this is illness by perception. I probably was always as clumsy as this. Maybe I never was good at reading aloud. Surely that bean in my groin is just my lymph nodes going about their business, tackling a cold I've had over the last few days. If you look for symptoms, you can find them. Every stumble and bump becomes something deeper. I no longer know what normal health is. Perhaps no cancer patient, even if they've been declared clear and call themselves a 'survivor', ever feels completely well again. They've been there, they've felt that vulnerability and fear. They will never look at a cold or a bump or a blemish in the same way again. Cancer eats away not just at your physical body, but your very sense of self.

I no longer talk of myself as a dying man though for the last three or four months that is exactly how I have felt. Instead, I begin to regard myself as someone living with long-term cancer, an illness that can never go away. It will inform everything that I do, everything that I am, even though for now it is not killing me. It justifies how I can look well on the outside, but explains why I continue to be plagued by fear, worry about feeling physically and mentally unwell.

There is one thing I cannot hide. I still want the seizures to go away, and was assured they would disappear once the medication was right. I go to see my new neurologist in London, the low-grade tumour expert who my private consultant recommended. There's a young man in the waiting room. He can't be more than 20 or 21. He's flanked on either side by his mum and dad. Dad's filling the silence with busy conversation: about motor racing, tennis, classic cars. Son tries to join in, but drifts away until Dad changes the subject and attracts him back. Mum is staring at her hands, messing with them to hide the shaking. Occasionally she smiles, laughs at her husband's observations. It's for her son's benefit. She's not really listening. Any talk is better than admitting where we are. Because we are in a brain tumour department, there can be only one reason he's here.

On my knees sits a blue plastic folder. It's two inches thick with reassurance. Letters of diagnosis, leaflets that say I'm looked after. Booklets that tell me what I'm going through, printouts with information I've downloaded from the internet. On his knees sits a single sheet of paper, empty but for today's date, a time and a doctor's name. He's dressed smartly for the occasion, he looks patient and fresh. I feel tired and jaded. I don't know the young man, but I feel like I've been where he is, and want to reach out. In six months time, he'll have a thick blue folder too. I want to introduce myself, I want to give him my number. I want to tell him it will all be alright. Though I know it won't be. Instead, I go to the toilet to cry.

When I return, the trio have gone and my name has been called. My new neurologist is relaxed and speaks with disarming humour. He's dismissive of my phantom symptoms: the imagined speech difficulties, the bumping into door frames. At the idea my stomach ulcer is anything to do with my brain tumour, he just smiles and shakes his head, amused. Even the tiredness, he says, would be down to the medication not the brain tumour. There's no reason to believe – given my type of tumour – anything at all would have changed in the months since my second MRI.

Even the seizures, he attempts to reassure me, are not necessarily an indication of tumour growth. It's just tumours doing what tumours do. The problem is, he says, that I'm not taking sufficient medication. I've only just reached the maximum dose of the drug I am on, and now it's time to introduce a new one. Most epileptics are on a mix of different drugs, but it takes time – his tone indicates a *long, long* time – to get a drug cocktail right.

"But the tumour is so big," I insist.

"Yes," he replies. "Which means it's been there a very long time. And you only get seizures on the bike. You're not even equal to where most people are when they are first diagnosed.

"Look," he says in his very most disarming, charming fashion while he scribbles out an illegible prescription for a new drug. "This type of tumour is measured in years, sometimes 15 years or more." My wife takes a note in capital letters. It's the biggest number we've been offered to date by a doctor. We shake hands, but I don't have time to thank him or make small talk on the way out. He's already speaking into his dictaphone, summarising our meeting.

For an hour or more we are reassured. I even feel embarrassed at having brought my imagined symptoms to his door. MRI imaging is what it is all about, that'll be the signifier that things have changed. Like looking on a radar for unfamiliar blips. The seizures are science, and science will deal with them. The rest could be anything: fear, stress, invention. And I know it's true. It's something we should try to hold on to.

Over the following weeks the seizures continue, but the other symptoms do seem to take a less aggressive pose. Most are still there, but they're more ambiguous. I remind myself to concentrate on trying to live with a brain tumour, rather than trying to die from it. The attitude fits well, but that doesn't mean it's always easy to wear.

My wife and I do a fundraising video for the Brain Tumour Charity. In it we talk about how difficult living with my condition is, particularly worries about the future. By the end of the filming session, all of us have tears in our eyes. But once the camera crew have left, I turn to my wife and say, "Do you think it was too much? Did we make it sound worse than it actually is?"

"Maybe," she replies. "Or maybe we're just getting used to it being like this."

I'm trying to understand cancer cookbooks. They sell enormously well: many dozens of them pop up on Amazon when you search for 'cancer'. The library bookshelves carry cancer cookbooks not only in the cooking section, but alongside medical textbooks and memoirs on those all-important cancer shelves. We're presented with the books offering the healing power of superfoods. The secret foods that will battle or beat our cancer. There are cookbooks stuffed with recipes that will, we're told, nourish the body and fight cancer cells. There are must-eat dishes to stave off cancer's approach, or to restore the body to its 'natural' state.

Cancer charities publish their own versions. The current bestselling cookbook in the UK is *The Royal Marsden Cancer Cookbook*, as if the touch of one of Europe's best-known cancer hospitals makes salads and soups somehow part of a serious medical intervention. I suspect the fundraising and marketing department at the Marsden played a bigger role in this book than the oncologists.

A cancer cookbook is just a cookbook. A cookbook with healthy, nourishing recipes and meals inside, sure. But there's nothing 'cancer' about it. Anyone could write a healthy cook book, full of diverse dishes low in salt and fat, including a rich mix from all the major food groups, and they too would have written a cancer cookbook. The most science has shown is that having a generally healthy diet and exercising regularly lowers our risk of getting cancer. It does not *prevent* cancer. It does not *cure* it.

There's not one superfood, not one ingredient, or food type, or even method for preparing food like juicing that has been proven to have cancer-preventing or cancer-battling properties. Some cancer cookbooks take a particular ingredient or food preparation method as their central theme: cumin, garlic, citrus, tomatoes, omega-3, juicing, antioxidants, chocolate, red wine. None of these has been scientifically proven to prevent, fight or beat cancer.

Eating one particular food or ingredient does not guarantee a life cancer-free, neither does avoiding a particular food. Gorging on a food not featured in a cancer cookbook does not mean you'll get the disease. Don't binge-eat on fast food and fatty red meat, don't wash down life with sugary drinks every day, don't smother food with salt, don't drink alcohol with everything. A little bit of all of these occasionally will do you little harm. A lot of them all the time will make you obese and unhealthy. It's the *obese and unhealthy* body bit that raises your risk of cancer, not the food that got you there. And if we're fat, unhealthy and alcoholic, consuming all the cumin we like won't redress the balance.

When we buy cancer cookbooks, what are we really buying? Hope? Certainty? A quick fix offering assurance that we've got our bases covered? Or worse, are we falling for a cynical marketing ploy? Attach the word 'cancer' to a run-of-the-mill healthy eating recipe book and double sales.

I guess cancer cookbooks follow the same pattern of most popular media coverage of cancer. If it helps to sell, then it's fair game. Media articles about alternative medicine treatments frequently come with overblown headlines: 'the cancer cure they don't want you to know about', 'revolutionary treatment', 'unexpected diet', 'miracle dad beats cancer'. The problem is there ends up being so much over-hyped news that it becomes difficult to tell what's true information about cancer, and what's hype promoted by someone trying to sell you something.

It takes a keen eye these days when searching for 'cancer

cure' or 'brain tumour' to turn up information that is truly helpful, compared with mere marketing for untested cures or preventions, or overblown tabloid news stories with no scientific backup.

Some cancer patients can separate the wheat from the chaff. Others are looking for the chaff in the first place. But for many, particularly those desperate for information about what's just happened to them, the best they can hope for is confusion and contradictory views. The worst is that they're attracted to a cure or treatment based on unproven or inconclusive information, but dressed up with power words like 'revolutionary', 'miracle' and 'ground-breaking'. That could prevent patients from getting the information they need or stop them pursuing a treatment pathway that may truly save their life.

It also means that when a real, truly revolutionary treatment is discovered or in development – right now, for example, cancer treatments based around specific gene signatures of tumours really *are* at an exciting stage – it's hard for the patient to determine whether this is the truth, or just another over-hyped news story using language that gets our pulses racing.

It confuses patients, it confuses those who give to cancer charities, and the confusion feeds the idea that in cancer effective treatment is just a case of whatever you fancy; that we have a huge range of equally valid available options. It also gives the impression that there are far more 'explosive' and 'revolutionary' developments than there really are. It foments the idea that our doctors and pharmaceutical companies are lying to us and trying to prevent us getting a taste of the 'exciting' and 'revolutionary' stuff going on. This stuff *does* exist in mainstream oncology, but it is rare. True progress is slow and precise. And the language used by science is far more measured, often more boring.

When a newspaper describes a 'pioneering new treatment developed by experimental doctors overseas' it could indeed be describing a real, scientific-based trial, governed by traditional medical testing procedures and ethics. But it could also mean some maverick doctor who claims to be able to cure cancer, but is working off-grid without medical oversight, without peer review or without using biologically plausible methods.

With the same words being used for two radically different types of trial, it's hard to know what to believe. In fact, particularly if a compelling human-interest story can be built in, the tendency is for sensationalist newspapers and TV to give the impression that alternative medicine is the better option, a bold, brave move in the face of institutionalised traditional medicine.

In February 2015, the UK tabloid newspaper the *Daily Mirror* covered the story of Kelly Logan where the headline read: *Mum refuses NHS cancer treatment to beat deadly disease with raw vegetable diet.* The story treated this as a brave stance: rather than submit to the hospital that wanted to 'pump me full of chemotherapy', she had decided to cure her breast cancer with a raw vegetable diet and exercise regime. The story came with pictures of Ms Logan surrounded by the supplements and fresh veggies she would be consuming.

Instead of listening to her doctor's recommendation, she decided to 'research alternative treatments online'. The story says that Kelly has taken her own life in her hands and 'wants others to do the same'. The journalist took an unquestioning approach to Ms Logan's self-healing, heralding her as a brave mum going against what's expected of her. It included only a short contribution, at the end of the article from a cancer charity telling readers, 'No alternative therapies have ever been proven to cure cancer or slow its growth.'

I face here the accusation of speaking ill of a mother who

had every right to decide for herself what treatment to have or not to have for cancer. I don't for a second deny her that right. But – and I mean this of all 'health gurus' who follow a similar path onto TV and into the newspapers to highlight alternative cures – by going public their story is no longer one of personal choice, it is one of leadership.

If going on TV or giving a newspaper interview influences the choices other people make, then that comes with a considerable amount of responsibility. I'm aware this is exactly what I am doing with this book. In its writing, I may well persuade some people to make more informed choices and to, for example, reject alternative treatments in favour of conventional medical treatment. I'm aware of the stakes, and I do not take that responsibility lightly.

TV news programmes, in the interests of balance, often present the alternative medicine debate in a way that gives alternative medicine and unproven treatments more credit than they are due. In one corner, a scientifically trained, fully accredited cancer researcher with years of oncological experience; in the other corner an alternative medicine practitioner who has none of their opponents' medical training and expertise (but may be more than a match in knowing how to manipulate a TV audience). Their opinions and treatments are presented as equally viable, simply as a choice between opposites. The viewer can make up their own mind. Like the cancer bookshelves, the programmes treat conventional treatment and alternative medicine as merely two sides of the same coin.

But this is wrong. These aren't two politicians presenting opposing points of view. In this kind of interview, the alternative practitioner's status and argument have been raised by being presented as an equal against the scientist. Meanwhile, the scientific opinion is reduced in its credibility, their work given comparative status with treatments that have never been proven, sometimes never even been tested.

The vast majority of medical work against cancer goes on quietly, methodically, slowly. Out of the spotlight, with only very significant and well-supported developments revealed to the media and, justly, carried as important news stories. There are far fewer significant and well-supported cancer developments going on in the alternative medical world. But a glance in the mainstream media would give the impression that 'explosive' discoveries are being made all the time.

We're led to believe, particularly if there's a bald child or a beautiful woman to photograph, that alternative approaches are equally valid players alongside mainstream medicine. American doctor Paul Offitt neatly sums up our tendency to turn more readily to quick-fix cancer books, rather than reasoned and scientifically sound ones, as well as the tendency for our various media to leap on the amazing and untrue stories. Writing in his critique of alternative medicine, *Killing Us Softly*, he observes the difference between the work of cancer survivor, diet book author and former actress Susan Somers, and physician, scientist, Rhodes scholar and writer Siddhartha Mukherjee, author of the history of cancer *The Emperor of All Maladies*:

"Nowhere in Somers's book do we learn about oncogenes and their products, and nowhere in Mukherjee's do we learn about coffee enemas and miracle diets. It's as if they were written in parallel universes. In Mukherjee's universe, drugs have to be science-based, thoroughly tested, and proven to work before they are licensed by the [Federal Drugs Administration (FDA)]. In Somers's universe, treatments aren't science-based, proven to work, or licensed by the FDA, they're promoted with testimonials and sold on websites. What is perhaps most disappointing is that television producers have consistently chosen Somers over Mukherjee to educate their viewers."

The British tabloids, like those across the rest of the world, continue to over-blow cancer stories. A single scientific discovery that an ingredient in the cacao plant might kill a cancer cell in a petri dish is blown up into a headline that 'chocolate cures cancer'. The tendency leads to the impossible conclusion that – according to media sources – various substances (chocolate, red wine, aspirin and many more) both cause cancer *and* prevent it. And we readers lap up story after story, failing to see either the contradiction or that a single experimental study in a lab can't be extrapolated to wider implications about whole food groups, treatments or cures. If it did, then 'fire kills cancer' would be a perfectly legitimate news story. Take a Bunsen burner to a petri dish full of cancer cells and you can be certain those cells will die. Many substances and actions do actually kill cancer cells; the problem is that they also kill normal cells. Only those treatments that do the former effectively without doing the latter quite so effectively become worth considering and testing as cancer treatments.

Even middlebrow newspapers in the UK know that cancer sells. *The Independent* newspaper ran a story in January 2015: "Eight-year-old girl Camilla Lisant suggests possible cancer treatment to her scientist father over the dinner table." It was a tale of a young girl suggesting to her cancer researcher father that he try to cure cancer with the same type of drugs they used to cure her sore throat. Dad went away to research it and did indeed find that antibiotics might help cure cancer.

It's a cute story, but it doesn't stand up to analysis. First, kids say all kinds of things at the dinner table. Before suggesting antibiotics, Camilla (as my kids have done) could have also suggested any number of other substances as a cure for cancer too: lemonade, grass, ice cream. But secondly, cancer scientists already do use antibiotics to fight cancer.

They're already regularly used in oncology. As the story reluctantly concludes, 'Dr Alan Worsley, Cancer Research UK's senior science communications officer, told *The Independent*: "Some antibiotics have been known to have anti-cancer effects since the 1960s and are a well-established part of cancer treatment today, alongside other chemotherapies."'

In other words, there is no story here. A girl suggested at the dinner table something would help fight cancer that we already know does. It's no more of a story than my daughter suggesting trains could carry more people if they had two floors and my having to tell her that such things already exist across Europe. We'd even been on one when she was a baby.

So the media can be irresponsible and poorly balanced when it comes to cancer – but this hardly qualifies as news. The point is that vulnerable, desperate people just diagnosed with cancer sometimes find it hard to access accurate information about their condition. They see TV shows deifying alternative therapy gurus or presenting them as of equal validity as science; or they read tabloid newspapers that talk of new 'sensational' or 'experimental' cures for cancer, and they believe them.

They believe them because we all want to believe in things that might help us. And the more people who pursue an untested, unproven alternative therapy, the more people will follow their lead. It sparks the beginning of a trend of people moving away from treatment that works, towards an 'equally valid' treatment that doesn't work and could even be dangerous.

The new normal

SO MY SECOND scan was clear: I remain a dying young man, but I am not dying yet. My neurologist has set me at ease about my phantom symptoms and pledged that with time we will deal with my seizures. They will stop and life will go on. It will never be the same as before diagnosis, but this is a new normal. And it doesn't look quite so bad as it has.

I'm still off work, knowing I don't want to go back to what I was doing. Not yet, maybe never. My daughter starts school in less than a month: I regard it with sorrow and joy in equal measure. She doesn't yet understand it's something she'll have to do for the next 14 years, nor what might happen in that time. Neither she nor I can turn back the clock.

Sarah runs a marathon, supporting the Brain Tumour Charity, and raises thousands of pounds from friends and family who find it a way to express sympathy for our situation. I write most mornings, but then take the afternoons off to suck in the sunshine; to eat picnics with my children, go for ice cream at the beach; to embark on long and labyrinthine cycle rides, clocking up the miles, exercising my body and exorcising my demons. I ride regularly on the weekends and in the evenings, in little races and minor time trials. I do OK, but the seizures are a constant barrier. I'm fitter than ever before. Is this what dying looks like? I've heard tales of cancer and brain tumours and this doesn't feel like any cancer I've ever known.

In the late summer, the children's grandparents kindly

offer to take them for the weekend allowing Sarah and I to go, unencumbered, for a long weekend in the picturesque Peak District National Park. The train journey is the first we've taken for a long time without the children in tow, and reminds us both how peaceful and liberating rail can be as a way to travel.

The short holiday is to enable us to talk: to take the luxury of beginning and ending a conversation without disruption; to allow our words to take us where they need to go without being disturbed by cries of needing the toilet or that a toy has been lost. The bed and breakfast we're staying in is wonderful, but it's the opportunity to be together and share our thoughts that is the real luxury.

We go on long walks, or amble around quaint villages, or sit by rivers and lakes taking in the scenery. We eat lemon drizzle cake offered by our host as we sit in her garden. We go out for unusually late meals without worrying about getting back for a babysitter. We spend time in bed, holding hands and looking at the ceiling and chatting in whispers.

There is no agenda. We just want to look at our lives through new eyes. My life is not in immediate danger. I am stable and could be for a very long time. It is our new normal. We need to process what has gone before. To look at the precipice my original diagnosis pushed us both towards, how we dealt with it and how we helped to bring each other back from the brink. Could it have been any different? Did we panic, or was our reaction normal? Did each of us – did I – do enough to be supportive?

But looking forward is more important than looking back. We remind ourselves that things are not what they were, that every decision we make for the future is now tainted. I'm writing a book on equal parenting and it feels like a legacy for my children. There are things to say about how they've been brought up so far, how I've tried to be a good and fair father, how I've tried to be a good husband, to be equal and to do what is right. When the book is finished, it will be my children's names I'll write in the front: an extended love letter for when I may not be around.

We talk about money: we need to write wills. It is something we should have done long ago, of course, but now we have no choice. But we also talk about my final care. What I think I want to happen when I can no longer decide for myself. When the time comes that I cannot express my wishes, I will long ago have lost everything that makes me me. There's resistance from Sarah, but understanding too.

I conclude there should be no hesitation on turning off any machine keeping me alive. I, as in *me*, won't be going anywhere. There won't be a *me*. My mind is just a connection of synapses and electrical pulses, adding up to feelings and hurt, love and opinion. Without life in the body, there is no mind. My light will be switched off, so the machine should be too.

We don't talk about the afterlife, but we do talk about the after-death. For me, the body will no longer matter to me once I am gone. We also talk about what is most rational after my death: to let me join the many millions of years of other organic bodies that simply lie down when they are dead to be absorbed into the ground. To become the foodstuff of other organic matter, to become soil, and rock and coal and water.

But we humans prefer to put our dead in boxes and throw flowers on top, to lower them into the ground and mark their position with concrete slabs. Or we draw the boxes into furnaces from which ashes are taken. They're offered to loved ones to scatter in memento, or to keep on their mantlepieces as if we're still there. As if those dirty, grey ashes will still be me. That the ashes of me carry some stronger significance than the simple fact that organic things are flammable.

Sarah and I talk about the simplest and most authentic

way to do what is expected of us: a memorial service with, more secretly perhaps, my long-dead body taken to a cold store somewhere where it will be slowly chopped at, sampled, perhaps displayed in chunks in university labs or under microscope slides, teaching children about muscles and blood, or for researchers to use to find out more about brain tumours. When I get home, I shall put all of this in writing, just to avoid any fuss.

We talk about our children and our daughter starting school, my little boy not too long behind her. It will be painful to have to let them go. Not to be able to hold onto them whenever I want to, to steal a hug when I'm feeling low. Shouldn't there be some special dispensation for people like me? Shouldn't I be allowed to hang onto my children like fret-blankets carried by babies, just in case I feel insecure? These are selfish thoughts, of course, so we talk more about how my daughter will settle in.

We talk about the school and how to tell the teachers about my condition. Erin knows that I am ill, but she doesn't yet know its severity or its dénouement. She wouldn't understand if we told her. But do the teachers need to know, in case over time she becomes distant, or worried, or things happen much quicker than we're led to expect? For the time being, we agree, there's nothing to say. No more than trying to predict my death from a road accident before it has happened. We'll let her first weeks and months at school be like they should be: those of just another little girl trying to find her place.

We talk about holidays and planning for the future: housing and work and ambitions. For too long, we have had our lives on hold. Too scared to look around the corner; staying still, crawled in a ball with our fingers in our ears. If we are to take the doctors at their word, then there is no reason to live like that. And that is a relief. We agree that we cannot plan with the assumption that the next six months – from scan to scan – are all we have to work with. We have to work and live and go on holidays and think about finances as if life will stretch on forever like we did before all of this began. If the worst happens, then we will deal with it when it comes. We cannot live our lives with death already on the horizon.

We will go back to work. We both crave the satisfaction and variety it brings. I will attempt to make my living from writing: books mainly, but perhaps some writing for charities again. I no longer want to be front of house: prancing around stages with PowerPoints and trick questions for the audience. I don't want to travel far from home, away from my wife and from my children, to do training or consultancy.

Writing won't make me any huge salary, but it will allow me to make the most of my family and to cycle when the sun is shining. Creating lines of words and having people read them and react to them is all I need from my work. It's what I have wanted all my life.

And then we speak about my seizures and my medication. It's clear that the drugs I'm taking have made no difference to the number or severity of the seizures I'm having. In fact, they're still becoming more frequent. We talk about my luck: that the seizures only come when I'm exercising. But then also my frustration that some of the very things that have helped me to feel sane over recent months are the very things that the seizures have disrupted. Why aren't the drugs working? For this, we have no strategy. There can be no plan or conclusion from our weekend in the Peak District. If the drugs are not yet working, there can be little I can do myself but try to adapt.

There is one thing I could do, I suppose. I could stop cycling, stop running. No exercise means no seizures, and that means no frustration. It's a question that has been asked of me by someone who ought to know me better: "Why not just stop cycling? You'll have to get good at chess instead."

It seems an obvious question, yet even the slightest thought reveals how insensitive, even offensive, it really is. For far over 10 years, cycling has been central to my world. This tumour is going to rob me of a lot of things over the next (as yet unknown) months and years. I'll gradually lose my ability to speak or communicate clearly. I'll get confused when I try to tell friends I love them or ask my children for a kiss. I'll gradually lose the use of my right arm and leg, followed by weakness down the right side, then the same on the left. I may not be able to hug, to hold hands. I'll lose the ability to stay awake for more than a couple of hours at a time. Then I won't be able to stay awake at all.

Right now, I can happily and safely climb onto my bike, point the front wheel down the road and just pedal. I can enjoy the freedom, satisfaction, fitness and fulfilment that it has brought me for more than a decade. Simply laying down the bike would be like simply laying down a leg, or a lung, or my kids, and leaving them behind. Could I willingly hang up my wheels before I have to?

My brother's lymphatic cancer was cured after nearly a year of treatment. He was declared all clear, the only remnants of his deadly illness being the marks on his chest that had been tattooed onto his skin to guide the radiotherapy machine. But the once-promising international middle distance runner never got his fitness back. He never quite achieved what his potential had been before cancer came to visit. It affected him deeply, inflicting a long-lasting hurt that long outlived the cancer that was cured.

Like for his running, giving up cycling would feel like a part of me has gone away. I would no longer be me. So while I still have a choice, my choice is to ride. I know how lucky I am to have that choice.

In the world of cancer, we have a problem with criticism. Criticism and cancer just don't go together, and so we self-censor. I know because I do it myself. Friends, relatives and others recommend miracle therapies and untested treatments and even though I know their words are rubbish, I don't tell them. I tread on eggshells around their suggestions, desperate not to offend. I say, 'well, I guess you never know,' even though I do. I don't tell them because at least they're doing something. At least they're trying. The shadow of cancer makes any attempt to help, however crass or insensitive or misleading, perfectly OK. I take the embarrassment, so they don't have to face it.

Against their brain tumour specialists' advice, Lucy Petagine and her family spend thousands of pounds of their own and others' money – freely donated – to send their child for Burzynski's unproven treatment in Texas because 'you have to try anything'. We call their actions full of brave hope, wish them luck, cry at their story. We don't tell them the truth. They've become immune from suspicions that their actions may be hasty, ill-judged, hysterical. We don't tell them they may be mistaken because haven't they been through enough?

The parents of Ashya King take their child out of a British hospital where he was already being treated for his brain tumour. They want faster treatment, more certainty, a treatment they've read about on the internet that their consultants have already said isn't appropriate for their child. We herald them for breaking free of the reins of bureaucracy. We praise them for getting one over the system. When their child is declared cured, we celebrate their actions. (Though doctors are sceptical of this cure.) Few dare say the parent's actions were selfish and crude, even dangerous for their son. Not worthy of praise. Because Mum and Dad always know best. A family is sprinkled with the fairy dust of cancer, which protects them from all criticism.

Jade Goody became an overnight success as a TV personality in the UK after appearing on the reality TV show *Big Brother*. It launched a TV career, a beauty product line and, five years later, a return to the Big Brother house, this time on the celebrity version. In that second visit, she was accused of racially bullying another contestant and became a nationally hated figure. For a time, she was the most unpopular TV personality in the country, with tabloids laying into her at every opportunity.

Then Jade Goody developed cervical cancer. She was declared terminally ill. Almost overnight, her reputation was transformed from racist bully into heroic cancer fighter. The TV and newspapers gave us daily updates. Celebrity magazines offered us visits insider her house and lengthy exclusive interviews from the dying woman. When she died, a number of newspapers – the ones who had vilified her before – ran full-colour supplements celebrating her life. Even the British prime minister at the time made a gushing statement about her death. Her funeral was broadcast on large screens outside the church and relayed live on Sky TV. Cancer had deified Jade Goody and placed her above criticism.

Most breast cancers occur in women over 50 and it is extremely rare in women under 40. Yet we say nothing when breast cancer charity fundraising billboards feature mainly attractive 20-something women, with targets emblazoned across tight T-shirted chests. As if by giving, we will blast the cancer away in the beautiful bosoms of only these gorgeous girls. Breast cancer only makes a newspaper story if it is a younger woman who gets it. The older women who are most at risk are all but invisible.

We daren't criticise the marketing strategies overtly because by doing so we may stand accused of threatening the income of charities that are, on our behalf and with our silent consent, fighting the bigger fight. Showing us the beautiful women to raise the money, then spending it preventing breast cancer among older women.

Cancer charities make strategic decisions to promote the stories of beautiful women with breast cancer, or child patients with leukaemia, to get the job done. They show us images of the pink bald head of a child dressed in teddy bear pyjamas. They know we'll dig deeper into our pockets for them, compared with for an old man in a dressing gown who will be hooked up to a drip for the rest of his life. We know charities do this. They know we know. But we don't raise an objection. We're not scared, we just don't want to break the spell. After all, the charities are getting the job done, they're trying their best. That's all that matters. Fighting cancer by whatever means necessary. Better the omertà than the empty piggy bank, right?

But some charities aren't even getting the job done. In the UK, there are nearly two dozen charities concentrating specifically on brain tumours. Some were set up in memory of someone who died and many have done little else since their establishment. They lie vacant and empty of funds on the Charities Register like floral memories of road victims that lie forgotten and rotting on carriageway verges.

A representative of one tiny brain tumour charity tells me: "All of our work is done by volunteers. We work from our kitchen table." And I nod along as if that's a good thing. I don't say what I think: that their charity should be closed down. That their effort and funds should be pooled into a larger brain tumour organisation. That way their work and expenditure won't be duplicated. The tiny sums they do raise will be made to work harder. Operating for free from a kitchen table may show altruism, but it also shows amateurism. It does cancer fundraising a disservice, not a favour.

But I don't say this because the charity still carries with it the memory of someone who died. Their very remembrance casts an aura around those who remain, protecting them from reproof. How many cancer charities were set up this way in a rushed desire to somehow remember, but now rest empty like an untended memorial? How far does our reluctance to criticise mean that energy, passion and grief is channelled away from cancer cure research, not towards it?

Do we self-censor to protect cancer patients themselves? Have those with cancer somehow earned the right to live in a cocoon of perfection simply because our DNA got wired up wrong? Have patients' families the right to special treatment? To be magically free from a critical comment because to disparage their actions, the tinctures they prepare, the beliefs they hold, would be to add to their grief?

What about those generously offering their advice to anyone who will listen? We too often take anything they say as acceptable, or at least don't tell them they're talking rubbish. Because they're trying? Doing something? In doing so, aren't we allowing potentially more damage to be done to avoid a personal feeling of discomfort?

Following our weekend in the Peak District, we do for a number of months live our new normality. My neurologist has increased my drugs dose. He still assures me that we will be able to bring my seizures in hand, to stop them from happening almost every time I run or go out on the bike. With the decisions we made in the Peak District about our future, we try to pursue what we have with renewed vigour.

A friend suggests I join him for a sponsored cross-country run. I decide it's just the type of thing I will start to say 'yes' to, instead of 'no – just in case'. The muddy run will be in early December, a freezing cold 10 miles through soaked soil, up hills, through streams and across rivers. My wife's father decides to join us, and together we start raising funds for the Brain Tumour Charity. It feels like something to look forward to, to work towards. It could even be fun.

But as the run approaches, I feel less sure. Not because of the mud and the cold. Those are things I would normally welcome. It's because I feel ever more tired and my seizures are becoming even more intense and regular. With the run intentionally sending competitors through freezing cold rivers and face-first into foot-deep mud to crawl under netting, it becomes clear that a seizure during the run would not just be inconvenient and disappointing, it might be dangerous. The week ahead of the event I spend so much time in bed or feeling dulled and morose that I finally decide I cannot do it. This kind of thing is no longer for me.

Sarah takes my place, and I go along to watch with the children, cheering our team along but feeling removed. I'm not for a second regretful that I'm not taking part. There are photos and videos of the day. Looking at them, I notice I am gaunt and skeletal, almost hunched over with pale and empty eyes sunk into wrangled sockets ringed with grey. I've been alive for 35 years. I look twice that age.

There's a Christmas tradition that marrying into my wife's family has brought with it. Normally, we spend Christmas at her parents' house, and then host New Year's Eve at our own. It's not that we stay up late: all of us are usually in bed by 10, having already counted down a fake Happy New Year for the children before tucking them up in bed.

For the family crowd, we serve piles of moules frites, prawns and oysters and crusty bread. Probably the most unsociable of the group, and possibly the slightly keener chef, it usually falls to me to do the majority of the cooking for the night while Sarah deals with drinks, laying the table and polite chat. I lock myself away in the kitchen and set about my work creating fumes of white wine, garlic and fish, smears of sour cream and crispy home-fried chips. Sarah dims the lights and the cameras roll as I, with aplomb, stride in: a tray piled up with bowls of moules and baskets heaped high with fries.

Just as I'm laying the first of the moules on the table, I feel a familiar creeping sensation from my right jaw. Soon, the right-hand side of my brain feels as if it is dropping away. My right arm feels slightly weak though I can see clearly that it is stable and strong holding a tray with the remaining bowls. I push the tray onto the table, scattering knives and forks. I dash from the room and for a reason I can't explain, go to my children's room and kneel on the floor.

I allow the seizure to come on in full. A blankness on the right-hand side, the feeling of my face pulling down on that side. I try to count and to speak to myself, but all that comes out is lumpy confused sounds. I'm fully awake, I know exactly what's happening. But there's nothing I can do to prevent it.

Over two minutes the seizure comes on, peaks, and then slowly dissipates. My father-in-law comes to check on me, I nod and my body language does what I intend it to: to ask him to give me some time. I kneel on the floor for five minutes. The seizure is long passed, but I need time to absorb the implications of what just happened. The feeling is only a familiar one of despair.

This is my first seizure that is 'unprovoked'. I have not been exercising: neither running or cycling. I had been calm, even celebratory as I brought the meal in for the family. It was a seizure entirely out of the blue, not only unwanted but also unexpected. As I look around my children's room, at the bright covers of their bunk beds, the luminous stars on the ceiling, the teddies and plastic figures scattered on the floor, I realise the implications could be huge.

From now on, New Year's Eve of all days, I could have a seizure at any time. Walking the kids to school. During dinner at a friend's house. Talking to a stranger. At the swimming baths. Ambling into a shop. I am no longer a man who can provoke seizures only by raising his heart rate and working his muscles. Now I have seizures any time and anywhere. I am an epileptic. It's not a label I like. Or at least not one I welcome added to the label of living with a brain tumour.

But there's more. There was a time when I had no seizures. There was a time when I only had seizures when I was pushing it very hard on the bike: sprinting for the line, or trying to chase down an escaped bunch. And even then only once a month or so. Then there was a time when I had cycling seizures more often, and then a time when I had seizures every time I climbed on the saddle, sometimes two or three. Then there became a time when I'd have a seizure every time I ran. Then there was a time when I felt so ill and vulnerable to seizures I couldn't even join an event with a friend to raise money for my own condition.

There has been a natural progression, there has been a change. And it's going in the wrong direction. My drugs are trying to chase it, but they just can't keep up. Without the drugs to temper the progression, would it have been even more rapid? Would the seizures have been even more deep?

Back at the table, I excuse myself for my rudeness. I've had a seizure, but it's gone now. Only my wife really knows the implications. We try not to allow it to dampen the evening's fun. I've only been gone for five minutes, my fries and bread roll are still warm. There's a pavlova for dessert, an easy pleaser. Afterwards, we dim the lights and the children watch with wonder as I light the indoor fireworks. I strike matches and hold them up to sparklers, and snakes and devils' tongues and glitter balls. What happens now, I think, if I have a seizure and have to drop the match, drop the sparkler? I put the thought out of my head.

I go to bed even earlier than I would normally. The seizure has shaken me and I feel I need to rest. To bring on tomorrow: a New Year, another new start? Pretend this year before hasn't even happened. In the middle of the night, I wake suddenly. Another seizure has begun to take over my body. I nudge Sarah and she wakes and immediately understands what is happening. She offers comfort, but mostly I just want her to see what happens. What it looks like from the outside. She's never seen me have a seizure before. This is something she'll have to get used to.

There's really little to see. My eyes feel vacant, but they're not. There is no twitching. I feel the right side of my body drop away, but there's no external change. I cannot speak. She laughs, but it is a kind and embarrassed giggle. One of comfort for me and for herself. We fall asleep soon afterwards, holding hands, as if it had been a silly dream.

On New Year's Day, I feel tired and allow myself to lie in. The day is quiet. But when night and sleep comes, I have two more seizures. The next night I have another two. Then another three the following night. For a week, the days are relatively clear, but the nights are punctuated by regular seizures that wake me from sleep. One night I have a record eight.

Now I do feel ill, never sleeping properly at night and tired, grumpy and bewildered during the day. And I watch as my wife takes the full burden upon her shoulders. The children have not yet gone back to pre-school or school. Every day they need to be clothed, fed, entertained and occupied. And every day, I'm like another she has to look after. I'm moody and needy, a walking zombie that can offer nothing to help. Some days I don't get dressed. If she's struggling to deal with the children and me, she doesn't say it. But dealing with the change in my health shows deep in the lines around her eyes.

I construct an email to my neurologist charting the change. I suggest he brings my next MRI forward from its planned date in March. I tell him I cannot sleep. I can barely function. Surely this is evidence of change, a symptom of acceleration that an MRI can only confirm as bad news.

His nurse emails me back. My doctor does not think an earlier MRI is necessary. She reminds me that my brain tumour, whatever it does, will do it slowly. Another six weeks will make no difference. But he will add another drug to my regime, one that's particularly effective for persistent seizures.

I begin taking the drug and soon my night-time seizures settle. First to perhaps one or two a night, then down to none. But day seizures take their place. This time the seizures are not deep, most often just a slight buzzing in my right jaw, a feeling of weakness in my right arm, the occasionally slip up of language.

The drugs have changed the nature of the seizures, but not their number. My wife and I begin to classify them: light, medium and deep. I tentatively get back on the bike. The deep, all-encompassing seizures that once had me leaping from the saddle and standing at the side of the road have almost entirely gone. Now I have light and medium seizures on the bike, neither so intense that I don't feel able to ride through them. For the first time, I start to feel like a cyclist again. Maybe soon I could even ride in a group. I let my imagination run wild: maybe I could race my bike this year? The thing holding me back would not be the seizures, but the fitness I've lost over the last six months. It's a cheering thought.

So much has changed in the last nine months, and each time we've been panicked by the change, then relaxed into it, then it's become just ordinary. I can't help but talk about the present as if it's always been like this. Once again, we're living a new normal. It's like the past experience of being in different health never happened. By the time I see my neurologist in the spring, my life with a regular mix of light, medium and occasional deep seizures already feels like old news.

How many times are alternative medicines, therapies and supplements promoted on the basis that they were traditionally used by ancient societies?

It's as if because a technique was used 3,000 years ago in China, or in ancient Egypt, or by native Americans, that particular treatment carries with it more credibility. If it was good enough for primitive Asian societies, then it's good enough for me.

But surely the opposite should be the case. That something was being done in the earliest days of civilisation to cure illnesses should make us more wary of those treatments, not keener to try them for ourselves.

Those ancient societies existed before we knew anything about the makeup of the body, about cells, about blood, about cancer, about the transfer of disease, the causes of illnesses. They didn't know the earth wasn't flat. Ancient societies may indeed have discovered a treatment that works for a particular complaint, but that doesn't mean all their other cures and treatments work too or that there was or is something magical about them.

Ancient practice is not always ancient wisdom. It can be modern wisdom too. If it turns out that something done by the Aztecs 1,500 years ago happens to be effective in treating a disease, then great: that's a treatment we can use today, irrespective of its origins. And indeed, we do use some techniques and drugs that ancient peoples used to treat illnesses.

For example, to treat flesh wounds ancient doctors used more or less same methods we do today. In India, medics were transferring flaps of skin from one part of the body to another more than 2,500 years ago. Around the same time the 'Father of Medicine', the Greek physician Hippocrates, pioneered the use of cauterising (burning) human tissue to seal off wounds. Ancient Egyptian doctors frequently used stitches and bandages to seal large cuts in the flesh.

One of the most celebrated ancient drugs is aspirin, a painkiller that stretches back thousands of years in use. Ancient Egyptians and Hippocrates refer to the painkilling effects of rubbing willow bark on injuries, the active ingredient being a forbear of – and still very similar to – the aspirin we use today to tackle pain and to prevent blood from clotting. Opium, derived from the poppy plant, is another ancient medicine used thousands of years ago and still employed today as a painkiller and as an anaesthetic. The foxglove plant has been used for hundreds of years as a medicine for heart conditions and again a derivative of its active ingredient is still used for certain heart patients.

These approaches and medicines are effective not because they are old or were used by wise and mysterious societies thousands of years ago. They're effective because they actually work. In more recent times, ancient medicine that works has been tested, analysed and refined according to modern knowledge about the body, medicines and disease, and for most we now know *why* they work too. Many ancient societies didn't know or were mistaken about why they worked, but they had success and so carried on.

But there are also a number of treatments, practices, cures and tinctures that ancient societies used and believed in that have now been shown not to work. Whatever they believed, the practitioners of 3,000 years ago were mistaken. Dung from various animals, fat from cats, fly droppings and even cooked mice are just a small selection of the range of remedies the Egyptian doctor would also administer as treatment to his patients.

Mainstream medicine is happy to reject the ancient ineffective treatments: they are an interesting window on past methods, but ultimately wrong in substance. In medicine, progress means the replacement of the old and ineffective, the unproven and dangerous, by the new and better, the proven and safer. Even some medical practices that are mainstream today will one day be regarded as quaint and naive. But the medical process can deal with that. It's how it's set up to continually try to improve. It's how progress in medicine works.

Yet alternative medicine seems to find it harder to let go of the past. Its practitioners continue to use the fact a treatment is ancient and mystical, that it has been practised for thousands of years, as sufficient proof that it must work.

On the menu offered by many alternative healers are ancient practices like Chinese cupping, chanting mantras, tracing life lines, aromatherapy, as well as sound, colour and crystal healing, amongst others. All are very old. None have any evidence to support them as medical interventions.

An unexpected development

AS NORMAL AS my life has become, after the changing of my seizures from occasional to frequent, I'm nervous as my spring MRI rolls round. It's been nearly a year since I was first diagnosed and this MRI feels significant. We're convinced this is the one that will be the one that will bring bad news. It is the first MRI to be taken at the National Hospital for Neurology and Neurosurgery. All my care has now been moved here. My original consultant had told me nothing was likely to happen to my tumour for years, perhaps many many years. But since that day, the seizures have just got worse and worse. He'd been wrong. Surely, something was happening in there.

We take our children out of school for the day and drop them at their grandparents so we can psyche ourselves up for the results meeting. We also want to spend as long as we need with the neurologist to talk about next steps – chemotherapy, radiotherapy – and take some time together to absorb the changes ahead. This doesn't feel like a results meeting you can prepare for, but it is one we can try to create a buffer around to make it easier to deal with.

The hospital is a beautiful old building on one side of Queen Square in central London. You have to duck behind the touristy restaurants and chain coffee shops to get there, through an alleyway which opens up onto a park in which patients, doctors and nurses sit in little clumps, eating packed lunches. My consultant's office is behind a newly built frontage, to the side of the main entrance. But once inside the modern glass gives way to the usual warren of grey and yellow NHS corridors, slow-moving lifts and forgotten staircases.

We check in at the front desk, squirting disinfectant onto our hands. We're directed to the lifts, but instead move around the back and go up the stairs to the first floor to arrive at the hospital's brain tumour department. There's a long corridor, off which neurologists, doctors and brain surgeons are breaking news, bad, good and somewhere in the middle. As we walk along it, we pass anxious patients sitting on plastic chairs outside each office, waiting their turn.

The corridor opens up into a tiny waiting room, a quarter of which is taken up by a reception area buried in towers of thick paper files. There's only a few empty chairs dotted around, so there ensues an uncomfortable shifting game as patients and family move around to allow my wife and I to sit together. Like the last time I visited this waiting room, I try hard not to look at other patients. They try hard not to look at me. When I do look, I see mostly people with nothing to indicate why they should be here. But there's always at least one, often two people in a wheelchair, or with radiation-burned faces and necks, or walking in with the help of a carer, unable to properly stand alone. We all watch them from the corners of our eyes, pretending to read the few magazines spread about the place or that we're writing urgent emails into our smartphones. It's a mixed emotion of empathy, guilt and self-interest. It's a gaze into a possible personal future.

When my name is called, my stomach lurches with sadness rather than nervousness. We're both ready for what the doctor is about to tell us. He welcomes me with a smile, his hand squeezing mine almost uncomfortably tight. For a moment, I think it must be good news. Impossible. Then I see his eyes. He's still registering who I am, putting the name on the folder under his arms with my face, taking a second to pull up my case from his memory. He must do this a dozen times a day. Why do I think he should remember me immediately? I'm just one of many.

"Ah, Gideon, welcome," he says. The light has gone on. "Please come this way." He presses the small of my back as I pass him in the corridor and enter his office. Inside, his nurse is sitting on the examining couch, swinging her legs. In the corner is a person I do not know.

"Gideon, how's the cycling?" the doctor asks. He's definitely got me now. "He's a bit keen on the bikes," he says, turning to the man in the corner and they laugh together. He introduces the other doctor; from what I can make out he's on an exchange programme with my neurologist, they're spending time checking each other's work and advising.

"Now, let's have a look at you," he says in the way a doctor does when they're about to examine your body. Only it's the inside of my head he wants, so he starts searching files on his computer looking for my latest MRIs to pull up on screen. "How have you been?" he says at the same time. Clearly he's not looked at my scan before he's invited me into his office. This will be the first time he's seen the new MRIs. Thirty seconds before, he was seeing his last patient out of the door.

We think our doctors only have us on their minds, all of the time. But really, we're only in their minds for the 10 or 20 minutes we're sitting in front of them. How many patients, how many brain tumours, does my neurologist see in a week?

I say, "Well, I've been fine. You know… about my seizures. They started coming when I'm not exercising, when I'm not on the bike. Then they started coming during the night, really deep." I hand him a graph my wife and I have constructed, charting my different seizures and the drugs I've been on. The line goes up and up.

"Wow, look at that," he says. He's impressed and amused

at the same time. He passes the graph to the other doctor, who nods with a similar smile before passing it to the nurse. Then he turns back to the pictures of my brain on his screen. The nurse knows me by now. She's received umpteen emails from me exploring the science and evidence on brain tumours. Something like this, she knows, is exactly what my wife and I would do.

"So," I say to the doctor, "you prescribed the new drug, and that's really helping. The seizures are still there, but they've been dampened down."

"Ah, yes, that's right," he says, swinging his chair round. "And the drugs are helping, that's good. So you're now on…"

I help him, listing the medication I take, and the doses.

"That's good," he says, adding that a combination of drugs is often the best way to control things. I look up to the scans on his computer screen, willing him to look in the same direction. He leans over his computer mouse and uses it to scroll up and down slices of my brain. He has my previous MRI scan from my local hospital on the left of his screen and my latest London scan on the right. He matches the slices up, so when he scrolls he can see the differences six months has made slice by slice.

"Well, all is good here as far as I can see, no notable change."

My wife and I breathe for the first time in the consultation. Perhaps he notices. "Yes, it's all stable as far as I can see."

How can you tell that? I think. By just looking at a grainy picture you're telling me nothing has changed? Then I think: you see many dozens of these pictures every week.

He looks down at the paper file in front of him. The radiographer's report says there's nothing to be concerned about, he tells me. There's a set of scans missing, that show the vascularity of the tumour – essentially how much blood it's taking up – but from the scan, he can see already that there's nothing extra the vascularity test will tell us.

Stable. Again.

"But what about the increase in seizures," I ask. "I don't understand. I thought it indicated the tumour was growing?"

That's true, he tells me. But the MRIs are a more reliable indicator. The seizures don't necessary match the change in a tumour. "They probably indicate a change in the metabolic environment of the tumour," he says. "We will have to do a biopsy or something some time." A biopsy or something. A biopsy is brain surgery. "But there's no change and no urgency here."

For now, he concludes, I should go away again. Come back in another six months, have another MRI scan, the process repeated once more. It'll be October before I'm back here again, I think to myself. Another lifetime away. He tweaks my prescription, adding another drug. He hands me a scribbled note to be taken downstairs to the pharmacy.

He rises from his chair. "So, we'll see you again in six months." He repeats his strong handshake, his smile this time betraying real happiness. I am one of his good patients. Keep up the good work. By the time we reach the door, my neurologist is already speaking into his dictaphone like last time, naming me and my hospital number. In three minutes, he'll be with another patient trying to place their name and face together, then pulling up pictures of their brain on his computer.

Sarah and I come out into the corridor, then head back down the stairs. It's only when we're on the outside of the modern facade that we stop for a moment to look at each other. We hug. Once again, against all expectations, I continue to be stable. I am free for another six months.

There's a little Indian canteen called Mama Thai that I know close to Liverpool Street station, towards the east end of

London. It's a tiny little place that review sites might call a 'hidden gem'. It's where I used to hide from the world when I wanted to be alone, yet surrounded by people on a Friday lunchtime to mark the end of another week. The food is incredible and embarrassingly cheap. I've been promising to show it to Sarah for years. With time to spare and good news to celebrate, I do exactly that.

So, what about God?

From the day of diagnosis, the world of religion, spirituality and God never once occurred to me as a solution – or even a mitigation – for my brain tumour. So many people seem to embrace or deepen their faith in the face of cancer, but to me the question never even arose. It wasn't a rejection of God. It just wasn't relevant. I've been an atheist for nearly two decades, so talk of God or the spiritual in relation to my condition would have been just so many words strung together, the sentences created having no meaning to me at all.

Until not long after university, I was a Quaker. It's a sect of Christianity, but within Quakerism the meaning of God was often drawn so widely that it seemed sometimes to lack any solidity at all. You could be a Christian Quaker, a Jewish Quaker, a Buddhist Quaker and even, it seemed, an atheist Quaker. With no central belief system or creeds, the line between being a Quaker and sitting around in a room in silence being 'open to the light' and sitting around in a room and doing not much at all became so blurred as to be invisible.

I do, however, have a degree in theology. But it wasn't devotional. It was a cold hard study of religion, religious texts and applying to religion the ideas of philosophy and the concepts of logic. Even as I continued attending Quaker Meetings (the Quakers' church services), I used to laugh along as my tutors told me nothing was more likely to destroy any faith I had than spending three years studying it in intricate detail. The logic and the analysis, the science of studying theology did exactly that. Religion, for me, became baseless. Mystical and interesting, sure, but also untrue.

So I never considered God as any part of the brain tumour equation. But religion reared large in some other people's response to my news. Particularly the notion of prayer. In personal conversations, in emails and in response to my blog, people offered to pray for me – or downright told me they'd be doing so. The offer of prayer was a very specific response to cancer and was a very specific offer to me as a patient. Whatever I felt about God or the concept of God, how was I supposed to feel about these offers?

What do religious people mean when they talk about prayer when it comes to cancer and brain tumours? The obvious answer is that prayer means asking God to change circumstances, petitioning God, asking God to intervene. But also there's an element of prayer that is worshipful: 'whatever you decide, thy will be done'. Whenever I've tried to talk to people of faith about these interpretations of prayer, there seems to be a clamming up. It's as if *that* isn't what prayer really is about. It's something different. A communing with God, a conversation perhaps, being *at one* with God. But the impression is that because I'm not a believer, it's something I couldn't understand. (Even with my degree in theology.)

Perhaps prayer has a different meaning for the religious than for the irreligious, and I can only go on what I know. And what I know is that religious people have made the concrete offer to pray to their God about my brain tumour, specifically to somehow help. But what does that help consist of? To make it go away? Make it less painful for my family? Make my death slower, or quicker? Whatever the purpose of prayer is, in the context of my brain tumour, there would have to be an element of *intervention* involved by God.

If praying isn't a call to intervene, then why pray for me? To talk to God *about* my tumour? To commune with God, because I won't do so myself? To be at one with God, while thinking about me and my tumour? If it is this kind of thing, then the kind offers made – however well intentioned – seem to me to carry no meaning. It may make the person who prays feel better or more secure, and that's OK, but it won't change the facts.

If what those who offer to pray for me do mean by prayer is more on the petitioning side and that they're asking God to change the situation – and this *is* what most people really mean – then that comes with its own particular set of logical leaps. The first is what philosophers have traditionally called 'the problem of evil'. If God knows that evil exists (by which is traditionally meant widespread disease, hunger, natural disasters, unending pain, undeserved death, and, of course, my brain tumour), then why doesn't He do something about it?

The traditional response is that God has given us humans free will, because to have free will and to allow us to respond to this evil is better than to have God control our actions all of the time. It might not look like it sometimes, but God has our best interest at heart. Free will was the greatest gift God could have offered.

But if this is what religious people believe, then where does prayer come into it? What does, 'I'll pray for Gideon and the cure of his brain tumour' mean? If God was going to cure my tumour, why allow it to be there in the first place? If we accept that God can intervene and will, if we pray hard enough, then why stop at my brain tumour? Even I (selfish, self-centred and arrogant as I am) would like to think if God was making the offer, I'd say, "If you're offering to intervene, please sort out malaria first. I'm way down the list."

What perhaps intrigues me even more is the physiological

intervention that the result of a successful prayer for my brain tumour would entail. My brain tumour is growing and this type of tumour will continue growing until it runs out of space and kills me. Or it will turn malignant first and start killing off other healthy cells in my brain. A prayer to save me would entail the tumour not following its natural progress that can only have been part of God's original intention. It would mean God making my tumour do the opposite of what it is *supposed* to do, biologically and/or against God's original intention.

Either way, it would mean my brain tumour has to stop growing, that it stops doing what it is DNA-bound to do, and it would mean that it doesn't turn malignant. There would need to be a point between my last MRI scan when it was growing and my next MRI scan sometime in the next six months when it stops doing anything. And then it would have to continue to not do anything for the rest of my life. I suppose this is the most plausible version of success when it comes to prayer, and all it takes is for God's creation to stop doing what God created it to do.

But there's a fly in the ointment. This would require a moment in time. A single point in which every brain tumour cell, but no other cell in my brain, suddenly decided to stop working. When would that be? The day of the prayer? A few days later?

Or is the prayer to make my brain tumour suddenly disappear? To cease to exist, to have disappeared from my brain and just no longer show up on the MRIs? This would require a bigger leap. I have the physical evidence of a four centimetre by four centimetre by five centimetre tumour (and growing) in the left-hand side of my brain. The proposal would be for that to just not be there on the next MRI. It would need history, effectively, to be reversed. Or perhaps a parallel universe where the tumour didn't exist, you'd never asked to pray for me and I wouldn't be writing these words.

The only other option is to argue that God will somehow intervene scientifically, through the natural order of things. That is to say, in the next few years God causes scientists to discover a cure for my cancer, or a medical development that slows its growth to a stop, or a better surgical technique, or something else, anything else medicinally, to stop my brain cancer from killing me.

This is where we get to the Quaker blurred line again. If this happens – and it's possible, though unlikely, that such a discovery will be made in my lifetime – how are we supposed to know that it was down to God, rather than the plod-plod-plodding along of science just doing its job? For religious people to claim the credit for something that could have happened anyway is no sort of religious claim at all. It's like the claim that a young baby pulled alive from the rubble of an earthquake is a 'miracle', while the dead bodies of hundreds of other young children line the crumbled streets.

Was the discovery of penicillin down to God? The sequencing of the human genome? If we credit God with all the 'good' discoveries in science, what about the 'bad' discoveries: the development of Zyklon B gas used in the Nazi death camps; nuclear warheads; addictive and harmful drugs? Francis Collins, one of the sequencers of the first human genome, argues that the wonder of DNA itself reveals God's existence and glory. Yet he fails to address why such a serious DNA-based disease as cancer shouldn't lead us to exactly the opposite conclusion.

Whether we can credit God with intervening in scientific developments or not is not quite the point. The point is at what point do we say: that scientific development would have happened anyway? And when do we say: that scientific development is purely down to someone praying for it to happen?

The latter fails the falsifiability test. If you believe God is intervening in ongoing scientific discoveries, what would it take to convince you otherwise? It's something that can neither be proven, nor disproven. Logically it's meaningless. We can agree to disagree. Either way, I'll live or die if and when the science allows it. So what role the prayer?

But there's also another niggle about those who responded to my news about my incurable terminal brain tumour by saying they would pray for me. It is that their immediate response is to tell me God will cure me. That somehow, because they have faith, they know better than scientists, and surgeons, and oncologists and years of hard information and evidence about my kind of tumour. That they have access to healing powers that I don't have because I don't believe in God.

The problem with the 'I'll pray for you' response is that it allows religious people to have their cake and eat it. To believe they're actually helping me in some way and to feel better because they are responding sympathetically and practically by actually doing *something*.

But that doing *something* amounts to asking God to change circumstances that God was, one way or another, at fault for creating in the first place. It feels like a hedging of bets: please change this, but if you don't, don't worry because I know it's all part of your wondrous, impenetrable wider plan which I can't understand. You're still worthy of my worship.

Prayer might feel like the only thing someone can do in the face of cancer, but it really isn't. Of course, it makes the person who prays feel better and that's great. We all need to find security in different ways. But if the religious want to do something specifically for me, or in response to my brain tumour, there are also a whole list of other things I could urge them to do.

Various cancer charities are desperate for funds, for people to volunteer, to take part in fundraising events. These are concrete and real *somethings* I can recommend and, from where I'm standing, will also get us closer to what I think the purpose of any offered prayer is: to save and prolong lives of those with brain tumours, and to reduce their suffering.

It's April and the brain tumour is gradually fading into the back of my life. We head off with some very good neighbours to the border of Oxfordshire and Wiltshire, to see his mum and to let our children play together. We enjoy walks, hospitality, space, emotional warmth and something amazing and delicious out of the oven every four hours. We're in one of those country villages where you can rarely get a decent mobile signal and we see that as a good thing. I take my bike, of course, and I head out early morning. The day is blustery, but not unduly cold.

I climb some of the steep hills to try to view the Uffington Horse. It's a vast sculpture cut into the chalky hillside by humans at least 3,000 years ago. Up a half-mile climb, I find only its foot. It's much better viewed from the air, but turning around to look at the geological ripples and dips I have just cycled across, the millions of years of geological features that history itself had carved out of the earth amaze me. Nature itself is so powerful and enduring, and very effective at highlighting my irrelevance.

Recently, I took my children to the Natural History Museum in London. If anything can put our human lives into perspective, it is looking at dinosaur bones. The sheer scale of time these beasts lived for, the awesome length between then and now. Most of the dinosaurs we see crowded onto single pages of a children's book would never have met each other. Even they lived millions of years apart. Time has stretched so far behind us. It will stretch so far in front once we've all gone.

Somewhere on the ride back to the village, my mobile

picks up a signal. When I arrive home, a message has been downloaded. It's from my neurologist: could I call him back first thing on Monday morning?

First thing. It's those two words and the tone he uses to say them that strikes me. I play the message to my wife. I play it to my friends. It could be nothing. But it could be something. A slight shadow has been cast over our time in the countryside. Instead of relaxing into the remaining day and night, I subtly pack bits and pieces, just so we can get off earlier, get home, and...

Well, what? Spend Sunday preparing for the Monday call? Tidy the house, as if someone important is coming to visit? Iron the children's uniforms and pack their school bags, as if the very act is going to make Monday morning come around more quickly? I try to relax, but a switch has been flipped. The countdown has begun.

When I saw my neurologist a month ago, everything had been just fine. We were prepared for the worst because my seizures had taken on such an aggressive and frequent nature. But the doctor had detected no growth in the tumour. I was stable. He had patted me on the back and told me to go home with some extra drugs because there was nothing to worry about.

When I'm put through to my neurologist, he doesn't hesitate. Do I remember that when he saw me in March, that there was a set of tests missing? These tests are called perfusion scans, he explains. They show the pathway of blood through the brain and tumour, and the uptake of blood by the different types of tissue. It can show angiogenesis he says: the building of blood vessels. He'd sent me away assuring me the MRI scans showed nothing to worry about so I shouldn't worry about the missing perfusion scans. His attitude was so casual, I'd forgotten about it a minute after he'd said it. He'd call me if there was something significant to say.

This was that call.

The missing scans have shown a significant uptake of blood in my brain tumour, a perfusion score of 4.8. I know not what that means, but the implication is that it's not good. I try to write down his words, but they're mostly technical. In between the jargon, I hear 'significant' and 'worrying' and 'abnormally high'.

"I think it's time to offer the opportunity to find out exactly what's going on in there," he concludes.

I take a moment to breathe. And then I reply: "Just for my clarity: are you offering me the choice between a biopsy, or hanging on for another six months to see how things go? Or are you advising me to have a biopsy right now?"

"Oh, I'm clearly saying you should have a biopsy," he says. "When we get a perfusion as high as 4.8 in this kind of tumour, we start to get twitchy."

'As high as', he says. In 'this kind of tumour'. Another set of casually spoken words that say more than I'd like them to. I've become important, someone to watch. I'm not just on the cusp of a question. I'm not even a slight worry. My blood vascularity in 'this type of tumour' is 'as high as this'. There's no doubt of its seriousness.

He says he'll refer me back to the brain surgeon I saw before. The one who referred me to him and who I thought I'd never see again. That brain surgeon will tell me about brain biopsies. They'll stick a computer-guided needle into my brain, into the areas of the tumour that are showing my high blood vascularity. They'll snip out some cells for testing, then they'll sew me back up. The aim of the operation is clear: to find out, once and for all, what kind of tumour I have. Because with a blood perfusion of 4.8, my low-grade brain tumour is no longer behaving like a low-grade brain tumour. Low grades transform into malignant ones; the question is when. And one of the early signs of transformation is high blood vascularity.

I go over the possible outcomes of the biopsy with my neurologist. It could be a low-grade oligodendroglioma (grade II) with an abnormally high blood perfusion. This would be OK news. It could be a high-grade oligodendroglioma (grade III), which is when a low-grade oligodendroglioma has transformed into a malignant one. This is less good news. Or it could be a high-grade astrocytoma (grade III). I ask my neurologist which of these was the one I least wanted to have. Astrocytoma is the name he repeats.

It is what it is, and the conversation finishes. We knew this was going to happen. My brain cancer is a progressive disease that can only move in one direction. Each is a slow step, and the hope is that each single step takes a long time. All indications are that I just took another step, and certainly a lot sooner than my results meeting last month indicated I might. Am I scared? No, not really. I already know where I'm headed, and there's something clarifying about moving forward. It's not good knowledge, but I guess it releases some of the pressure. I'm not sure I've made peace with the information, but I've come to an understanding.

Am I sad? Yes, of course. I look at my young kids playing, or making jokes at the dinner table, and they don't really have a clue what's happening. I listen to the deep sadness in my wife's sighs, see the welling up as she answers questions from her friends about how I'm doing. I'm sad for my family, for the inevitable blankness, the empty chair. My concern for them far outweighs any feeling of sorrow I have for myself.

But mostly, right now, I'm intrigued. If things go badly, I'll come out of hospital and straight into radiotherapy, perhaps chemotherapy too. Life in another new direction. I can't say I relish the thought of the treatment. Nor of the honest assessment that for me they will only ever be more steps, never a solution. I can't say I'm enamoured by the idea that with radiotherapy, I'll only get one six-week cycle because the brain can only take a certain amount. It's my trump card, and I may well have to play it soon.

The biopsy will offer more than just clarity about what my brain tumour is up to. It will also offer the genetic signature of my tumour. We'll know for the first time whether the DNA in the tumour cells carries specific genetic strings that could make treatment more effective for me. The tumour's genes can have a significant impact on life expectancy. So a biopsy will offer me a clearer picture of what the future may hold. It is this kind of clarity I crave.

I go to enjoy a pasta lunch with my family. Then I speak calmly with my wife about what the doctor had said, we make a cup of tea and sit closely together to watch our kids play for a while. Then I go back to my office, intending to work. The biopsy referral could take many weeks. There's nothing to do to prepare. Still, I start to search the web for strange brain tumours with strange names. I end up looking at a paper written by my own neurologist about high tumour vascularity and its correlation with malignant transformation. I don't like what I read.

I look up from the screen and see the sun threatening to fall over the horizon. So I close the laptop and take my bike out instead. A lap of the reservoir, on past the jam factory at Tiptree and back along a winding country road, finishing over one of my favourite rises which at its top offers an inspiring vista of the sunset over the water and the Essex countryside beyond. What else could I do?

Cancer doesn't care about you.

Cancer isn't something going wrong in our cells or the DNA floating within. There's no evil motivation. Or at least, not on the part of the cells or the DNA. It's DNA doing what DNA is supposed to do. As far as the DNA is concerned, it's getting it absolutely spot on. Only DNA doesn't get concerned. It's just instructions. If good is doing what you're supposed to do and doing it well then cancer is good.

Under the microscope, cancer comes with no personality. No malignant or benign intent. It's just numbers, digits, dots on a graph. DNA molecular bases. Protein pathways. Molecules fitting into each other, or failing to fit.

Cancer happens because the DNA inside cells changes. It can be caused to change by the things we do or the environment around us, or from natural mutations we've inherited. But most frequently it changes for no reason at all. Just random stuff going on in our cells. That's at the very heart of what DNA does. Sometimes nothing happens. Most often the disrupted DNA fades away, engulfed by cells that hold their sequence. Sometimes it doesn't and the disruption grows.

Some like to tell us every one of our cells has cancer. It scares us into buying unproven therapies, supplements and treatments to prevent the cancer taking over. Cash in exchange for security. But they're saying no more than that our cells have the potential to evolve. Without DNA disruption, there would be no development. Without DNA mutation, there would be no evolution. There would be no us. I would look just like you, you just like me. We'd all be less than single cell amoebas, floating in the primordial gloop.

People tell us cancer is unnatural, even evil. That their remedies will return our bodies to their 'natural' state. But cancer is the most natural thing in the world. It's exactly how we're supposed to work. Without the natural mechanisms behind cancer, our hair and fingernails wouldn't grow, our body wouldn't heal. Cancer is just as natural and good as our ability to create new life.

To impose words like 'go wrong' or 'bad cell' are understandable ways for humans to deal with it, but cancer isn't anything of the sort. A cancer cell with mutated DNA isn't a cell gone wrong at all. The DNA is working perfectly. Just because it's not convenient for us doesn't make it a bad process. Cancer isn't resentful of our fight, grateful if we fail. When we fight cancer, when we battle it, we should remember that we're battling something that's only evil in our own eyes.

What is cancer? The World Health Organization defines it as a group of around 100 diseases characterised by the uncontrolled growth of abnormal cells. These cells grow beyond their usual boundaries, multiplying out of control. In some cancers, they invade adjoining parts of the body and spread to other organs.

That's a pretty clear, but also a very wide definition. It is probably one of the reasons why cancer seems so ubiquitous. Everything from a deadly brain tumour, via a blood lymphoma, to a next to harmless basal cell carcinoma skin cancer or an almost entirely curable testicular cancer, all fall under the same catch-all name. It makes us feel vulnerable and scared, fearing the cancer that is all around us.

But the truth is that all cancers are not the same. Many are not the death sentence we assume them to be, and which historically they may have once been. When Cancer Research UK says that around one in two of us will get cancer it feels like a scary statistic. And it's one some will use to claim cancer is an evil epidemic, on the precipice of overcoming us unless we take natural supplements or radically change the world in which we live.

But as the charity acknowledges itself, the statistic is the opposite of a scare story. In a sense, the one-in-two prevalence of cancer is good news. It demonstrates that we're all living longer, but those extra years necessarily bring with them their own risk of cancer diagnosis. The biggest risk factor for cancer is getting old. But now when that diagnosis comes, there's far more that can be done about it than in the past.

As individuals affected by our own deadly cancer, it seems hard to take the good news because we have the wrong sort of cancer, with the wrong prognosis. To us, cancer is too big, all encompassing and disastrous. But as a complete population of humans, cancer boils down to a simple sum: the certainty of many extra years of better quality life for most people, in exchange for a nominally small extra risk of cancer per person's (now increased) lifetime. As a population of humans, we don't hesitate to accept those odds.

The statistics show that we know more about cancer. We detect it better. We have better screening programmes. We make diagnoses quicker. More people may be being diagnosed, but the progress of medicine means it often doesn't bring with it the dire implications it once did. In that sense, science's 'war' against cancer is actually going in our favour. We may never succeed fully, but we are 'winning'. Far more people are surviving better detected cancer than ever before. And we do know how to save yet more lives from cancer, such as those incidences caused by human behaviour. We know we should stop smoking, reduce drinking, avoid obesity. The fault is not the science, but the lack of humans actually doing much in response to what the science is telling us.

Like with cancer, the science doesn't care about us. But we certainly should care more about the science.

The great cancer conspiracy

I ASSUME THE biopsy is going to take weeks to organise, but my seizures intervene to bring it forward. Despite the new drugs prescribed by my neurologist at the stable-but-it-ended-up-not-quite-stable MRI results meeting a month before, my seizures continue to come light, but they come more frequently than ever. I put an average seizure count at about seven or eight a day for the last week or so, but this week has been different. On Monday, I have 14 seizures. Yesterday, I stopped counting at 20. Today, after six seizures in an hour, my wife gives my neurologist a call.

"That's not normal," he says when she manages to get hold of him. "He needs to come into hospital, tonight if possible." This hospital is about an hour and a half's journey from where we live. I know that even if I set off now, at 7 p.m., I won't get there until 9 p.m. Add another hour to be admitted and by 10 p.m. do I really expect a neurologist would still be around to come and see me? My wife tells him I will come in the morning, and he says to double the dose of my most powerful drug in the meantime.

The next day I drop my kids off at school without any fuss, then head into London with my wife. There begins a farcical hospital to-ing and fro-ing, a moving in and out of waiting rooms, waiting in corridors, and squeezing into offices without any chairs. I arrive at the National Hospital for Neurology and Neurosurgery at 11.30am without a clue about

151

what to expect though hoping for at least some intervention to bring my seizures under control. I'm passed around the hospital: from neurology to surgery and back again, for the next six hours. The biggest surprise comes at lunchtime. A phone call from the surgery department, asking me for details so they can arrange the biopsy I'll be having tomorrow.

"Biopsy?" I say. "No one said anything about a biopsy."

I know I am due to have one. But that was supposed to be later. After I've discussed it with a consultant. Given it some thought. Weighed up the risks. I want to know things about brain surgery before I have it. Things like: what really happens during a brain biopsy? What are the side effects? Will I come out able to speak or move? What are the chances of not coming out alive?

I am eventually sent up to the ward at 5 p.m., and the surgical registrar tries to book me in for the night and my biopsy the next morning. I shake my head and simply say 'no'. I explain that no one had even described what the biopsy would entail, let alone given me a chance to talk to my family about its implications. I don't want to get caught up in a tsunami of frantic action that would see me going under anaesthetic and the surgeon's knife within hours, without my properly understanding what was going on and why. It was the seizures I'd come to hospital to be treated for.

The registrar then does explain the biopsy procedure, the difficulties of taking a sample of my particular tumour. I would likely come out of it with temporary loss of some motor and speech functions. In up to three percent of cases, those functions never come back. There could be other complications. There's a one percent chance that I'll die.

But I still refuse to be bumped straight into the operation the next morning. It would be taking the phrase 'sleep on it' a little too literally. All I can think about are my children. I've not said anything to them. Just dropped them off at school as if it was a normal day. I'd not shared a moment with them. Not taken a last look in their eyes, or kissed their soft foreheads just in case. The next time they see me I could be in a pretty bad state. My head bandaged and possibly unable to speak. It would be cruel. Unexpected. Unacceptable.

Instead, the consultant books me in to stay the night for monitoring. They will take some blood, monitor my seizures and revisit my drugs doses. They will arrange the biopsy the following week if I decide to go ahead. I take off my shoes, get onto the bed and 15 minutes later my neurologist arrives. He is full of profuse apologies. He hadn't made it clear that by 'get you into hospital' he actually meant 'give you a biopsy'. He does still advise I stay and have the operation tomorrow (you might as well now you're here, is the general gist) but no, it is not urgent. No, it won't stop the seizures. And yes, of course, it is my choice whether to have it or not.

He then tells me what we have all really known for the last few weeks: he strongly suspects my tumour has turned malignant. But if I want to wait, then there's no need to stay in the hospital tonight.

So I go home to see my children's bright faces and listen to their chatter about what toys they'd brought with them to their grandparents' house. I kiss them and hug them, and ask questions about what they've done today. I *will* have the biopsy, I know it is worth the risks. I'll call tomorrow to arrange the operation for a week or two's time. But I know, without a single doubt, I have done the right thing today.

I like both my GP and my neurologist. Apart from their general friendliness, I think the reason I like them so much is that they've always been honest with me. When I first reported my seizures to my family doctor, he told me he genuinely didn't know what was up with me, but he wasn't happy and so wanted to refer me.

My neurologist is happy to reply to some of my more demanding questions (How long have I got? What does that new blob on my MRI show? Is this new symptom significant?) that he simply doesn't know the answer. There's so much in brain tumours that has not been pinned down and every patient is different. If he gave me confident and certain answers to every question, then there's a good argument that I should be less trusting of him, not more.

Proponents of alternative medicine like to point to the faults in the conventional medical system. If you think alternative medicine has problems, well just look at the corruption, failures, deaths, negligence and mistakes of conventional medicine. They're hardly perfect.

And they're right. I've been lucky. My experience of the UK National Health Service (NHS), especially in regard to my brain tumour, has been generally good. Not always perfect, but eight out of ten isn't bad. But some have been failed. Some have felt mistreated. Some have been criminally neglected. Some people's health problems have been misdiagnosed or missed in a negligent rather than an accidental way.

Drug companies too have routinely hidden research, falsified data, inflated costs or found ways of protecting their products at the expense of patients. Their behaviour has sometimes not just been on the edge of neglectful and selfish, it has been criminal. Conventional medicine and pharmaceutical companies, and the researchers and scientists, absolutely should be criticised for these failings. And crucially, they should be held accountable.

To some extent, many would argue, they are held to account. There are overseeing bodies, medical councils, ethics committees and peer reviews. Yet still, there are monumental failures. Some very good books, journalists and critiques expose their failings in intricate detail. I urge anybody to turn to them to be enlightened and outraged in equal measure.

But here's the thing. If the area of conventional medicine is sometimes poor, and medical research has some significant weaknesses and failures, it does not for one moment mean that alternative medicine is better, that it should be free from critique, or that the conventions of mainstream science should not apply to it.

Just because mainstream medicine is far from perfect does not mean we should reject the whole system and embrace alternative treatments without question. To believe that mainstream medicine, its methods and conventions, has nothing to tell us about non-conventional medicine is an irrational mistake. But it's one that proponents of alternative medicine use to push their own agenda: that alternative therapies and techniques are somehow special and should be excluded from the scientific method.

In his oncology and psychology textbook *The Cancer Experience*, Roy B Sessions, a US leading head and neck cancer surgeon, argues that cancer patients' relationships with their doctors has changed over recent years. These days, he argues, patients see their cancer doctors as just one of a number of choices to make when they are diagnosed. Their advice, born of years of study and professional experience, is just another option from which patients can pick and choose.

This is the commodification of medicine. And it is partly the result of the proliferation of cancer diet and prevention books, alternative medicine techniques and self-declared cancer experts that have claimed we should put everything presented to us on an equal footing. As one breast cancer patient, who refused to have the surgery, chemotherapy and radiotherapy that could have saved her life, put it to a newspaper, "I felt doctors were biased towards conventional treatment."

To which one might answer, 'Yes, your doctors were in

favour of conventional treatment. That's because conventional treatment is likely to work and a diet of raw vegetables almost certainly won't.' A doctor's job is to prescribe what's most likely to work. There was never any bias at play.

At the same time, we have an irrational expectation of our doctors to know everything and give us immediate and correct answers on demand. If they don't know the answers to every question we have, then they're not doing their job properly and we should, therefore, go somewhere else to get the answers we want to hear.

We ask too much of our doctors, and even charity campaign groups are at fault for leaving too much blame at doctors' doors when things go wrong. If we go to our family doctors with symptoms, and they send us away with an antibiotic prescription, we may or may not get better. If we get better, do we sing their praises? Or do we just think: well, the doctor was only doing their job?

But what if we don't get better? What if it turns out we have cancer? Suddenly our doctor has failed us because they've 'missed' our killer disease. They didn't spot it. They're incompetent. They deserve vengeance, deserve to be sued. In some people's eyes, they're part of the cancer industrial context that *wants* us to die from cancer.

My local family doctor works in a surgery that serves my village and the three or four other little villages close by. He told me after my diagnosis he'd only ever seen one other case of a brain tumour and it was very different to mine. When I first went to him, he could have had any reaction. He could have sent me home, telling me I'd been pushing it too hard on the bike. He could have said to give it two weeks with these tablets. He could have said I was imagining it. Doctors do these things all the time; sometimes they're right and sometimes they're wrong. What my doctor did was send me to a stroke clinic, thinking this was the best way to discover what was going on.

Did he think I'd had a stroke? I don't think so. He could just as well have sent me to the heart and chest department. Did he think I had a brain tumour? I doubt it very much. He just didn't know. He did what any family doctor is supposed to do. Make an initial assessment, then refer me on if he thought it was necessary.

Did he misdiagnose me? Absolutely not. If he'd sent me home, would he have neglectfully failed to spot my brain cancer? Would he have let me down? No, of course not. In the brain tumour community, I hear all the time that local doctors didn't spot that people had brain tumours first or second time. Patients had been sent away. Or in hospitals, doctors blamed migraines on stress or on sinus trouble. Vision and hearing problems had been explained by earlier problems with eyes and ears, rather than the unknown brain tumour lurking deep inside. And there's blame. There's a baying for vengeance that the doctors didn't get it right. That they are worthy of our fury.

But mostly doctors aren't to blame. The brain tumour is there and doctors – without that knowledge – do their best with the time, budget and medical ability they have to make the best guess at what our problem might be. We criticise them for sending cancer patients home with one breath, but with the next for over-subscribing medication or sending relatively healthy patients to hospital just in case.

I am not advocating a blind trust in doctors and oncologists. Doctors do get it wrong, and the medical establishment is far from perfect. But I also that know doctors are human beings and can make mistakes. That's why I got a second opinion about my brain tumour. I wanted to wait, I wanted to read up, I wanted to check and double check. I exercised scepticism and criticism. I took time to think for myself.

But if we exercise scepticism and doubt about medically trained doctors, oncology and conventional medicine, then we should subject alternative medicine to at least the same level of doubt and scrutiny. In fact, I would argue alternative medicine deserves far more doubt because it self-consciously puts itself outside conventional medicine that has been proven by time and experience to, mostly but not always, get it right.

My doctor came to see me not long after my diagnosis. He wanted to see how I was; how well the family was keeping it together. He also wanted to apologise: he said he should have sent me straight for an MRI. Looking back, with the benefit of his reading up further on brain tumours, he thought he probably should have suspected a brain tumour or at least some serious lesion in my brain. But I don't blame him at all. He'd executed his role exactly to the letter. If he'd sent me away for six months with an urge to keep an eye on it, I hope I would have come to exactly the same conclusion.

A rational examination of the medical establishment does give us reason to be mistrustful, or at least to recognise doctors don't always get it right. By their very nature, family doctors aren't going to get it right first time, every time. They have a necessarily shallow knowledge of a broad number of things. Their ideal position is to be able to reassure, sort, deal with what they can, and refer on anything they can't pin down. That is a proper understanding of the doctor's role, and even a realistic assessment of what expert consultants (including oncologists) can achieve, based on the knowledge they have. They're not merely one of a number of choices we can pick and choose from like a buffet of health options. They're the first port of call, and we should respect their role better.

But what about the multinational pharmaceutical companies, the so-called Big Pharma that proponents of alternative medicine like to blame for a cancer epidemic many of them say these big companies have created? There's no doubt once again that there is reason to be sceptical about the motivations and behaviour of Big Pharma. There are reasons to be more than cautious.

The history of private sector pharmacology is one of hidden studies, unpublished results, undue influence and corrupt practice. There is reason for anger at Big Pharma, not only for letting us down but also for creating doubt about the drugs and academic disciplines that control lives and deaths, that influence doctors' and consultants' advice about our health.

But there's an important distinction here. Big Pharma may sometimes have exploited or distorted the scientific method, but they're not the method itself. Since the 17th century, all scientific testing has been based on the same basic norms: the prediction of results, creating experiments to test whether your prediction is correct, ensuring the experiments aren't influenced by yourself or other biases, receiving the results, interpreting them and deciphering whether they matched your prediction or whether you should make a different prediction next time. Vitally, the method demands the whole lot is made available for criticism and interpretation by other professionals (peer review) to ensure your predictions and experiments weren't flawed. The method is not perfect, but it's as close to brilliant as anyone has ever got.

With the addition of open reporting, scientific journals, meta-analysis of data and ongoing replication of clinical tests with new methodology, the medical process is close to robust. Medical trials of drugs, theories, treatments, diagnosis and much more are all based on this close-to-sound scientific method. We shouldn't doubt the system, only learn from the abuse that Big Pharma has sometimes subjected it to. What should make us angry is that by abusing the system Big Pharma has worn down trust in it. They have made us believe it is broken and flawed when it is not.

This provides an easy excuse for those who don't want to submit their alternative techniques and cures to testing. Because the methodology is broken, they say, we can't use it to test alternative medicine's claims.

But a call to scepticism of mainstream medicine necessarily demands we subject alternative medicine to the same scepticism. If, despite all the checks and balances, Big Pharma has got away with so much over the years to skew data and behave badly, then how much more sceptical should we be of alternative medicine that has no – and never has had any – independent checks and balances?

Critics of the 'the great cancer conspiracy' use science and statistics when it suits them, but quickly abandon them when discussing their own treatments. They are quick to claim chemotherapy causes or doesn't prevent cancer death, and to quote official statistics of the numbers which traditional medicine has failed to save. They bring up official medical statistics for cancer death increases, and drugs that were approved but then withdrawn because they were shown to be ineffective or harmful.

But alternative treatment proponents cannot have it both ways. If they wish to use science and the medicine testing protocol as a standard against which to argue conventional techniques aren't good enough, then they must subject their own medicines or techniques to the same protocols.

If alternative medicine proponents tell us that chemotherapy doesn't work we should indeed look at chemotherapy. Ask questions. Look at the data. The thousands of results, and meta-analysis, and research about chemo's success and failures. But we should also ask the same questions of alternative medicine.

And when we play this game, in every case the balance falls very heavily in favour of conventional medicine instead of alternative treatments. In every single case, conventional medicines – the much-hated surgery, chemotherapy and radiotherapy – outstrip non-conventional treatments hands down. The two are not even in the same ball park. And what's more, the data about conventional treatments is right there, available to read for most practitioners (and increasingly for the public too). It can be compared and used to make big decisions. Alternative medicine provides no such data, no such comparison.

The pernicious and consistent claim laid at the door of Big Pharma by alternative medicine is this: Big Pharma either does not want to find a cure for cancer, or it already has the cure but is keeping it secret. Similar to this, Big Pharma won't test alternative medicine treatments because alternative medicine is 'natural' and they can't patent natural products and so cannot make a profit from them. As Chris Woollhams writes, "Big Pharma is just not interested; there's no profit in natural compounds. They can't be patented."

In worst cases, the accusation is that Big Pharma has governments, industry and doctors in their pockets, paying them hush money to keep the secret so they can continue to make money from cancer drugs. This is not a joke. One of the most widespread alternative cancer treatments (and one of the ones that makes the most money) is Gerson Therapy. In the video Cancer is Curable NOW! Charlotte Gerson, founder of the Gerson Institute set up to promote her father's treatment, makes the really quite incredible accusation about Big Pharma sitting on a cure for cancer:

"It would ruin the economy. Billions of dollars. And we live in a medical dictatorship. Big Pharma, the huge pharmaceutical companies that make billions from cancer, have everybody in their pocket. From the President, down to the Senator's Representative. Everybody gets paid."

It's an accusation I've heard dozens of times when I've tried to argue that alternative medicine has not been proven to work. Big Pharma won't invest in alternative medicine because they won't make any money from it. They don't want a cure because they make so much from existing cancer treatments that don't really work either.

But where is the basis for this astounding claim? Intuition or 'Big Pharma must be doing this because cancer hasn't been cured' is simply not good enough. What research has been done on this accusation? What papers have been published? What examples can be given? What legal cases have taken place? Where is even the smallest shred of evidence that Big Pharma behaves in this way?

An examination of these accusations reveals they are surely incorrect, if not ridiculous. Big Pharma does want to find a cure for cancer. Surely it is desperate to do so, given the money involved. In fact, Big Pharma has made, and continues to make, great strides towards amazing advances in cancer treatments and cures. The published paperwork does not point to Big Pharma trying to close down cancer treatment, it clearly shows Big Pharma trumpeting every minute development it makes.

Big Pharma has been involved in many of the major discoveries regarding cancer in the last generation, and they're already supplying – and making money from – drugs and treatments that help to cure cancer and destroy tumours.

Avastin, created by drugs company Roche, is one of the biggest and most effective cancer drugs in recent times. It has helped to save many patients diagnosed with colorectal cancer, and is used to prevent blood vessel growth in tumours for many types of cancers – including certain types of brain tumours. That doesn't sound much like Big Pharma trying not to find a cure, nor much like Big Pharma trying to keep secret the cures it has already developed.

Big Pharma is already doing very well indeed out of cancer, and it knows that the better it is able to tackle cancer the more money it will make. If a Big Pharma company could develop an anti-cancer vaccine, or perfect a process like gene therapy that could better target and control tumour growth, it would be heralded the world over. Their scientists would be held aloft by millions of cancer patients and their families. Governments would pay the hugest amounts.

The accusation that Big Pharma doesn't invest in alternative medicine because it can't patent natural cures is also just as ridiculous. Firstly, alternative medicine practitioners do a decent job of making money out of their own natural cures, don't they? Secondly, companies the world over make billions every year selling us things that are naturally occurring and can't be patented. Indeed, many companies make millions selling to us one of the most abundant substances on earth. When was the last time you drank from a plastic bottle of water? Water is natural, non-patentable and so ubiquitous that it falls from the sky. Yet companies sell many billions of litres of fresh water to us every year. Most natural and health food stores sell bottles of water too.

Companies sell things to us all the time that can't be stamped with intellectual property. What they are selling is convenience, brand, style, a sense of identity. However 'natural' or abundant a cure for cancer may be, you can bet a Big Pharma company will find a way to package it and sell it to us. Just as other companies do with milk and smoothies and potatoes and salt and firewood and sand.

The idea that natural things can't be sold to make a profit is negated by the very existence of natural health food stores. Each is jammed full of naturally occurring ingredients, neatly and conveniently packed into foods and supplements and bottles. Indeed, the multibillion homeopathy industry is based on the very idea of packaging up literally nothing but water's supposed memory of a molecule, and then selling it to willing customers.

It's also worth noting that many of the large natural supplement companies and brands are actually owned by Big Pharma corporations. Bayer, which produces proven cancer drugs, also owns natural supplement and vitamin brands One A Day and Redoxon. Pfizer, which has developed effective breast cancer medication, owns the world's best-selling multivitamin Centrum and calcium supplement Caltrate. So Big Pharma already *is* successfully selling us supplements that are natural and non-patentable. And they're most often selling them to those who claim to reject Big Pharma.

Note too that large pharmaceutical companies (many of whom also do a mean business in genetic modification of crops) have become adept at taking natural substances, tweaking them ever so slightly at a genetic level, to turn once naturally occurring substances into owned intellectual property. In other words, they have the knowledge, the wherewithal and the lawyers to take previously non-patentable natural substances and to go ahead and patent them anyway, before selling them for huge profits. That a cancer 'cure' is natural would certainly not be seen by Big Pharma as an unbreachable barrier to making money out of it.

The final logical destruction of the idea that Big Pharma either doesn't want to cure cancer, or already knows how to but is keeping it secret, is simply the ludicrousness of such an enormous conspiracy taking place. The fact is that Big Pharma companies are owned, run and staffed by human beings. People. People who get cancer. Hundreds of thousands of people work in the industry and among them some will get cancer. Their mums will get cancer. Their children will get cancer. Their partners will get cancer. Their friends will get cancer.

It is not a credible suggestion that a parent of a child who is dying slowly and painfully from cancer would keep secret the knowledge he or she has: that cancer is curable. Is a father really going to allow his own child to die for the sake of a wage packet?

Even those right at the top of Big Pharma. The men and women in suits, sitting in dark rooms supposedly controlling the cancer industrial complex, along with the presidents and prime ministers who are in their pay; even they get cancer. Facing their potential death, is loyalty to the company so strong that they'll go to their deathbeds without uttering a word about how they really could have been saved? Is it credible that thousands of scientists are keeping the cure for cancer secret? That not one single rogue scientist has ever broken ranks and told the world about the big conspiracy? Not even one who's been sacked from their job or is disgruntled with their boss? Not one who's even posted anonymously on a whistleblower website?

Arguably, a fair proportion of people went into cancer research, cancer drugs and treatment research exactly because they were affected by cancer one way or another. Their very employment in the cancer sector was motivated by finding a cure. Do they suddenly turn silent when they discover one already exists, but they can't tell anyone because it's natural and can't be patented?

That Big Pharma is hiding or doesn't want to cure cancer is the conspiracy theory of conspiracy theories. It's very utterance takes the public to be complete fools while acting as a platform for us to be sold 'natural' treatments. Those who claim Big Pharma doesn't want to find a cure for cancer, or won't research natural cures, or already has the cure but is keeping it secret, do the alternative medicine scene no favours at all. It destroys whatever credibility alternative medicine might ever have been able to claim.

A brain biopsy

BY DEGREES THEY make you feel ill, even if you're not yet sick.

I arrive at the hospital in jeans and a T-shirt, a rucksack slung over my shoulder, a bag with snacks for later. It's as if I'm checking into a hotel. Actually, I say at the ward reception desk, "Oh, hi, just me, you know, checking in." They show me to my bed, and a nurse comes along and takes my blood pressure, measures my oxygen levels, and sticks a thermometer in my ear. Just checking my 'obs', she says. Have you got the wrong person, I think? I've not actually had anything done to me yet.

Are you allergic to anything? Any medical conditions we should know about? Apart from the brain tumour? Ha ha. Oh, well, actually there is this kidney thing I had when a child. And the appendectomy. The stomach ulcer. My brother's cancer. A life of illnesses come back to haunt me, scrawled down on a chart at the end of my bed in ballpoint pen.

Then the metamorphosis begins. It starts, of course, with the white band. One on the wrist, then another on the ankle. Slow step by slow step, my gradual acquisition of the accoutrements of sickness reminds me that all is not quite right.

"That'll be it for the night," says the nurse. "You won't see anyone else."

It's only about 6 p.m., and my wife is still here. I'm in a

ward with six other guys, some reading, some sleeping, a few grunting and grumbling in pain. Fresh sheets, a big screen TV for us all to share, my own little cupboard, a little reading lamp. I could get used to all this. A bed in central London would normally cost you a fortune. We break out the snacks.

A doctor turns up at 9-ish. He's on his rounds. He takes some blood. He asks me about any allergies (again) and checks me over, shining a torch in my eyes. *Hold my hands, now push against them, now pull. Very good. Now to the side, push right arm, now push left. OK, now the feet.* He has a white plastic stick with a rubber doughnut on the end and sets about banging different parts of my body to see whether my reactions are intact. They are. Like I say, nothing has been done to me yet.

Do I know my name? My date of birth? Where I am? What's the date today? "That's all for tonight," he says over his shoulder. "Someone will be round to see you in the morning."

My wife leaves and now I'm starting to feel like I ought to be sicker. Maybe I'm letting someone down. I'm an impostor in this place of ill people. I'll blend in better, I decide, if I lose the jeans and pull on my pyjamas. Twenty minutes later, a surgeon comes up. He's dressed in blue gowns and sports a surgical cap. Whose brain have you been inside today?

He explains the procedure. Tomorrow morning they'll send me down for an MRI scan. That'll help guide the surgeons as they drill a hole in my head and use a computer-guided needle to take pieces of the tumour for analysis. He goes over the risks again: the death, the permanent disablement, the stuff that's been going round and round and round in my head for the last week. From midnight, I'm not to eat. From 6 a.m. I must not drink. He finishes off by drawing a big red arrow in marker on the left side of my neck, pointing up. In case someone gets confused and tries to do brain surgery on my backside.

He's reassuring, but with all these tests and warnings and instructions, I'm feeling a bit more like I'm starting to fit in here. But I'm in good hands. Though he's clear about the risks, he seems so relaxed about the operation. I'm a pretty routine gig around these parts. As he leaves, he just about manages to say no one else will come and see me tonight when a new nurse pops her head around the curtain. Time for my 'obs'.

This nurse is no messing. Stern. Matronly. She does my blood pressure, my oxygen levels, my temperature. She hands me one of those gowns that leave little to the imagination, and some tight socks to prevent DVT. I need to change my own pyjamas for these, she instructs. I will, I promise, next time I get up to go to the loo. She looks sceptical, then spies the book by my side, waiting to be read just as soon as I stop getting disturbed. You should be going to sleep, she says, and turns out my light.

At 11 p.m. some poor guy has just been brought in: he's suffering, obviously struggling. He cries out in pain, gurgles through the tubes trying to keep his airways open. I drift off, but at 3 a.m. the nurse – the one who told me I should be getting some sleep – wakes me. She has to put on some stickers so the surgeons can guide where the needle will go. I sit up in bed, and she plasters my face and head with a dozen circular pads. Then she pulls from her pocket a green magic marker and colours in the centre of each circle. The whole process takes no more than three minutes.

"Now, get some sleep," she says.

It's 6 a.m. and a new nurse calls around. He wants to check I've taken my epilepsy drugs. Six is the start of the day in a hospital. There are no lie-ins here. People are milling around, orderlies are throwing open curtains. The twice-daily cleaning of the wards has already begun.

I get just a sniff of other people's breakfasts before a

porter comes to take me down for my MRI scan. Of course, I'm still in my pyjamas, even now resisting my last induction to the world of the sick. He stands and watches as I don my gown, finally jettisoning anything that makes me feel I may not belong here. He has a wheelchair, but I say I'd rather walk. We go through ward after ward, through corridors, down stairs, past the reception desk and into the MRI department.

By the time I return from MRI, my wife has been to my bay and left some cycling magazines and a newspaper on my bed. Just as I'm beginning to browse, my surgeon comes up to see me. He's so relaxed, he practically gets into bed next to me, "So, you know what we're going to do?" he says. "And you know about the risks? OK, great. It's going to be just fine. We're still working on the guy before you, but once we've got him closed up, we'll get you down there. A couple of hours. See you in a bit."

My wife comes up 10 minutes later. She's sheepishly clutching a cup of coffee. She knows if there's one thing I'd love right now after 10 hours nil by mouth – even more than an armful of cycling magazines – it's the half-litre of steaming hot Americano she's bought for herself.

Our good friend arrives. She'll sit with my wife while I'm downstairs. It's great to see her, but I feel guilty because we've got a long wait until I go down. I'm just about to say this when a porter arrives at the end of my bed, "Come on then, you're up."

Everything then happens in a flash. All feelings of nervousness or reticence have gone. This is happening, it's happening right now. There isn't a chance to think.

The three of us troop down to theatre; I'm handed over to the anaesthetist, who goes over the consent forms with me again. I kiss my friend. I kiss my wife.

Within minutes, I'm lying on a thin theatre bed in the anaesthesia room, ever so slightly flirting with the anaesthetist as she pushes a syringe into my arm.

Then I'm gone.

I knew her. I'm sure our paths have crossed. I read her story in a newspaper and followed it up on the internet. I can't place her name, Kate Gross, but there's something in her smile. The cheeks and bright eyes. So familiar.

I tried to think back 15 years. We went to the same university at the same time. But we were in different colleges. If I did know her, it can't have been that well. But reading her article in the paper, the posts on her blog, I get the impression we were into the same causes, shared political values. So maybe our paths crossed in student politics. Or later, when she set up her own non-governmental organisation, perhaps we met as I moved around the charity sector too. Or maybe there's nothing. Maybe I never knew her at all.

Kate Gross died on Christmas Day 2014, aged 36, from incurable bowel cancer. She was one year younger than me. She left behind a husband and two boys, neither of them yet the seven years of my oldest daughter. I read her final thoughts in the newspaper, her messages to her boys. The clarity of her thought, the sensitivity of her voice, the calm understanding of her own death, her hopes for her family, the final words for her loved ones. My heart breaks.

I follow the links from her article and find her blog. I read what she calls 'the inevitable page about how it started'. On it I read about her frequently irritable bowel – 'irritable and annoying'. I can imagine her laughing as she writes, and I'm jealous at her clever turn of phrase. She returned from one of her frequent trips to Africa, visiting one of her charity projects. She'd been sick and disorientated at the airport. Probably just a bug she'd picked up. Less than 24 hours later, surgeons were opening up her colon, trying to remove each of the tumours that had made it their home. But the cancer came back. Her bowels again. Then her lungs, her bones, her blood.

In a particularly memorable blog post, she writes about acceptance. The rational retreat from cancer treatment that had done what it could, into palliative care. She lived her last weeks writing words for her boys to read and hold in their hands, a remembrance of her and what she was like. A treasured book they'll still read again and again, even when they're far older than the age she was when she died.

I read her pages and I feel love and grief and sorrow. For her, for her sons, for the charity and its staff that she left behind, for the loss of those smiling eyes. I probably didn't know her, but she's become part of my life, part of my own past and part of my future.

I finish her blog, the parting thoughts she wanted to leave to the world and those who loved her, for those whose lives she'd touched. Inspired, I scroll down to look at the comments left in remembrance of her.

And then I become angry. The first comment, the very first contribution, is not one of sympathy or wisdom or even one of solidarity.

"Have you heard about the healing power of raw foods?" it asks. It leaves a YouTube link to a video about one plant or another that will cure the cancer she has just written that there is no hope of her recovering from.

How could you? How dare you? Do you think you are helping? Do you think you are offering support, reaching out? Or did you not even bother to read the words under which you are now sharing your miracle cure? Did you merely see an opportunity to press the same old nonsense, dressed up as something natural, clean, smooth and life-giving? Did you think your words would be consoling for others reading this blog? That your comment would be something her family members would enjoy reading, something they might offer up at her memorial service, as they thanked everyone for their kind messages left online?

I don't know how she felt about that post, about the countless others who offered her other miraculous cures or healthy, natural ways to beat cancer. I do know that for each of the other comments offered on her blog, she responded in person. A thank you for their thoughts. A little advice. A sympathetic thought offered back, dismissing her own terrible situation. But I notice that the post about 'the healing power of raw foods' goes without comment. Other 'miracle cure' posts generously left by well-wishers also go without a note or response. Yet they sit there.

She was stronger than me. Perhaps more open-minded, or at least more thoughtful for others reading her blog, thinking that even if she didn't get anything out of suggestions, that perhaps someone else would.

I know I'm not so open-minded or giving. When someone makes similar points under my own blog, I simply delete them. They languish in the trash can I've dumped them in as soon as they arrive. That little symbol shaped like a dustbin is the most I offer to such posts, dragging and dropping them angrily, selfishly, before signing out.

Maybe I didn't know Kate Gross, the one with the smiling eyes and now motherless children. I wish I had. Perhaps she had something to teach me about tolerance and humility.

If you have ever had a general anaesthetic, you'll know it's nothing like being asleep. You're out for hours and hours, but when you eventually wake up you have no sense that even a second has passed. It's like you've blinked. I'm lying, looking up at the ceiling. There are people milling around and I take a moment to check myself over. Fingers: right hand, one, two, three, four, five; now left. Toes, the same. I count to ten out loud. As I whisper I can hear my voice. It sounds normal. The registrar comes, the same guy from last night. He welcomes me back, checks my vitals, gets me to do the pushing/pulling thing. He asks me my name, the date, where I am. All faculties apparently intact. I drop back off, and he comes back ten minutes later and repeats the whole thing.

Sometime soon, my wife arrives and they wheel me upstairs. Inexplicably, I'm already lying in my hospital bed and they reverse me back into my parking space. Standing alongside, there are two more familiar faces, both beaming: the friend who has been with my wife for the five hours I've been under, and her husband who has just arrived from work. Their welcome, their smiles, their simply being there, brings a tear to my eye.

We hug and kiss and laugh and take photos. We tell inappropriate jokes about the tubes going in and out of my body. I'm still sky high on the drugs, but it feels like we're the funniest comedians in town.

Sometime later – it could have been ten minutes, it could have been two hours – my friends have gone and another great friend arrives. He brings more cycling magazines and flowers. Though I'm falling in and out of sleep as we speak, it's amazing to have him there. More photos for the album. An hour later, he leaves. My wife follows not long after.

I spend the rest of the evening and night intermittently sleeping, being woken up every two hours for my 'obs', and unsuccessfully trying to pee into a cardboard container. I am obliged, it appears, to prove to the nurse that my body is processing fluids properly. Gone 3 a.m. she's almost threatening that if I don't pee soon, she'll have to stick another needle into my arm to get more fluids going round. The threat does its job, and when the flow does come there's plenty of it.

The operation, I am led to understand, went well. No complications, no problems. It took longer than expected, but only because the surgeons needed to send tissues down to pathology to ensure they got some tumour. But they did get some, and in just over a week's time I'll find out what they got. There's a hole in my skull, with two inches of skin sewn back up over the top. Unexpectedly, there are staples in either side of my head where the surgeons screwed my head in place to prevent it moving during the operation.

As I'm tucking into breakfast the next morning, another friend comes. He makes more fun of me because I'm sitting there like a whale with a blow hole in my head. At least I can drink the coffee my wife brings up for us both. Then, after some paperwork, I'm released back into the buzz of a city going about its business. I leave the hospital wearing a cycling cap on top of my bloodied bandage. We make our way back on public transport to the suburbs, alongside the bustling city folk calling it a day at 3 p.m. and streaming into the pubs to enjoy the sun.

Arriving home, my children seem not to have missed me one bit. Nor are they interested in the plaster or the staples in my head. Still, I'm surprised how good I'm feeling. I only came out of surgery about 18 hours ago. It's as if nothing has happened. And it feels good that way.

But the next day I have a headache. A big one.

I'm back in the historical building on Queen Square, behind the modern glass facade. Two weeks ago, I was downstairs somewhere. Deep in the bowels of the National Hospital for Neurology and Neurosurgery, my head being drilled and probed to pick out parts of my brain. I can't say I'm delighted to be back here because it's results day. My surgeon will tell me what the biopsy found: the type of brain tumour I have. In doing so, it feels like he'll be mapping in more detail the rest of my life. Particularly how far that life might stretch.

We're in another part of the hospital this time. It's more modern. This waiting room has a snack machine and a huge flat-screen TV. There's a presentation about the hospital on loop. The chairs are padded and comfortable, bright green. The whole waiting room has a matching colour scheme, as if patients have been consulted about what would make them more comfortable as they wait for the most important results of their life. For me, the toilets are too close to the waiting room. I'd like further to walk, so time is easier to waste as I wait for my turn to hear the news.

We try to read magazines, to chat, to browse more cancer leaflets and patient feedback forms. Nothing works, so I watch the people going by. There's an older man with a large plaster covering most of his head. He's surrounded by family members, who hold hands and occasionally pat and hug him. He's not quite there. My cancer nurse passes, recognises me and stops to say hello. She's not seeing me today, just on her way somewhere else. If she knows what we're about to hear, she doesn't let on.

Eventually, we're shown through to a modern consultation suite. Like the waiting room, it has co-ordinated furniture, paintings on the walls above little plastic bottles of hand sanitiser and emergency oxygen equipment. In the chair today is my registrar brain surgeon, the second in command during my biopsy two weeks ago. He's the one who pushed and pulled against my hands, asked me to count to ten, if I could remember my name and knew the date.

I have, he says, an oligodendroglioma brain tumour. I roll the word around my mouth like a mint. He smiles as I try it. This, he tells me, is good news. It's all relative: I know an oligo is still an incurable brain tumour. It just goes about its business slightly slower than the alternatives. Again, I want to thank him for delivering the good news. But there's more.

The biopsy recovered eight tiny slices of my tumour, where it was showing signs of likely malignancy. Every piece recovered was grade II tumour, not grade III. There's no proof, as yet, that my tumour has turned malignant. It's the best outcome we could have hoped for. I've come out healthy, with no obvious neurological problems. If anything, my seizures have calmed down. Yesterday was the first day since New Year when I didn't have one at all. The tumour turns out to be the very much better end of the bad ones. And it's *probably* still low-grade: a grade II tumour rather than a grade III.

Probably. That's as certain as we can be. This is a subtle but important issue to understand when it comes to medical tests. And it's this kind of thing that proponents of alternative treatments confuse when it comes to medicine. My biopsy has not proven that my tumour is definitely grade II. Nor has it proven that it is not a grade III tumour. All it has proven is that the slivers of tumour the needle took away were all grade II, so there is definitely some grade II parts of tumour in there. It's quite possible there's grade III tumour in there too. The biopsy might have missed those bits.

When alternative medicine proponents claim that medicine and science has never proven that, say, wheatgrass doesn't cure cancer, they've been asking the wrong question. Scientists aren't interested in what doesn't work, they're interested in what does. It may be possible that wheatgrass does treat cancer, but no experiment has ever proven this. That's not proof that it doesn't cure cancer, but it's a fairly clear indication. All we can do is make a pretty good supposition.

My biopsy didn't find any grade III tumour cells, but my biopsy didn't test each of the millions of cells in my tumour. That there were no grade III cells in my tumour is simply unprovable. That none of the eight samples contained grade III cells gives an impression, and allows a rational and reasonably-made supposition.

I ought to be delighted to have come out of the biopsy remaining a grade II. But in real life, in real medicine, things are never as simple as that. I was, my doctor tells me, the subject of quite some debate among the medical team looking at my biopsy results and my latest perfusion MRI this morning. On the scan, my tumour shows clear signs of taking on more blood in certain areas. Add that to my massive increase of seizure activity this year and there's reason for concern. The final medical consensus was that we *should* proceed, albeit grudgingly, as if I *do* have a grade III tumour.

Having a grade III brain tumour changes the picture. It means I probably need to start treatment. The watch-and-wait period, with only MRI scans every six months, is over. It's time for something else. And that something else is probably radiotherapy and chemotherapy. Not tomorrow morning, probably not even this month. No one is going to hand me a blister of chemo tablets on my way out of the hospital. But the game has definitely changed.

It is what we expected when we walked into the hospital this morning. The seizure changes surely couldn't be just bad luck. Those missing vascularity test results, and the hesitation in my neurologist's voice when he told me about them: that wasn't imagined.

The doctor sends me away with an appointment to see an oncologist. It is she who will plan my treatment and oversee it. By the time I see her, she will also have further important information about my tumour. The samples have been sent for genetic testing. Researchers are looking to see if the tumour's cells have a certain set of genes missing from their DNA. If they do, that will be good news. Patients with oligodendroglioma tumours that have the so-called 1p/19q and IDH1 'deletions' tend to have a longer life expectancy, and they are more likely to respond to radiotherapy and chemotherapy.

This is where cancer is these days. Specific chains of genetic bases in our DNA, and their influence on our treatment and chances of recovery, survival or keeping the cancer at bay. It's molecular. Drilled down to DNA molecules, proteins, nucleotides. Minuscule chemical pathways allowing molecules in and out of the walls of mitochondrial cells. It makes the idea of 'whole-body healing', 'treating the whole self' and 'maintaining a cancer prevention terrain' nothing less than an ignorant and wilfully blind embarrassment when it comes to cancer. Even a very basic understanding of the role of genetics in cancer shows most alternative medicine has no idea at all what it's dealing with.

As always, I leave the hospital with more questions than answers. What does my tumour's genetic signature say? Will it be chemo and radio? Chemo or radio? Radio then chemo? Chemo then radio? Will starting it sooner rather than later really make a difference to the overall outlook? If so, by how much? What does 'soon' or 'later' or even 'outlook' mean in this context: weeks? Months? Years? If there's no certainty how long I'm going to live right now then what meaning does 'extending my life' even have? I'd only be extending it theoretically, a mental somersault simply adding one lack of clarity on top of another.

My oncology meetings will happen in the next month or so. Some questions I know will be answered. Others, there are no answers to.

What makes you an expert? There's often a guru mentality in cancer where those with no qualifications or recognised track record freely declare themselves experts in the subject and begin to proffer their views for others to hear.

Countless books on cancer, particularly those of a 'natural' and alternative medicine bent, see the author claim to be an expert. They've spent 10 years researching cancer, they've dedicated their life to alternative medicine approaches, they've dealt with hundreds of patients, dozens have left testimonies on their websites.

I have a brain tumour that will become a cancer. I've known about it for nearly four years, and spent many months of those on the internet and in libraries absorbing information, talking to fellow patients and doctors. Does that make me an expert? Should you listen to me more carefully than a surgeon or a brain doctor, simply because I have the condition we're talking about and they don't?

I've written a book about my specific type of tumour. I've worked with a brain cancer charity on their marketing materials, leaflets and videos. To some extent, brain cancer has become my life. But I'm not an expert. I have knowledge. Pub quiz knowledge. But I've not begun to scratch the surface. I can't call trumps on anyone else for my expertise, much less medical doctors.

Yet there are cancer prevention and cure books written entirely on the basis that the author themselves, or their mum, or their daughter, had cancer. The author set off on a mission to 'discover everything I could about the disease'.

Being a patient or a patient's family member doesn't make someone an expert. And it certainly doesn't mean they have the right to trash trained doctors, and brain surgeons, and anyone who happens to be paid by a pharmaceutical company. Nor does it allow self-proclaimed experts to accuse real experts of hiding from the public the secrets they supposedly hold about cancer prevention, or accuse them of having cures they don't want the public to know about.

Laura Bond, author of *Mum's NOT Having Chemo*, decided to become a health and cancer expert when her mum was diagnosed with ovarian cancer. They wanted to avoid conventional treatment and pursue alternative therapies instead. She is now a self-declared 'health coach'.

Her book highlights Dr Burzynski's treatment for brain tumours and plugs his promotional video. She calls him 'a

Texan doctor curing universally fatal brain tumours' but doesn't mention at all, let alone on the same page, that his treatment is not only unproven, but one of the most controversial in cancer worldwide. Another controversial cancer treatment is Gerson therapy, another central theme of Laura Bond's book, which receives uncritical promotion.

It takes one single Google search for the Burzynski controversy to come up. The second search result on him is a Wikipedia page that goes into extensive detail about criticism of his treatment, and reveals that it has never been proven to work. Google search results four, five, six and seven are all about the controversy surrounding the doctor.

Anyone who claims to have spent years dedicated to researching cancer cures and recommends Burzynski, but does not include any reference at all to the controversy surrounding him, the Federal Drug Agency action against him, or the simple non-proof of his work is either a terrible researcher or is choosing to omit this arguably vital information.

The same pattern emerges when self-declared 'experts' or 'health coaches', who reckon they've researched their subject thoroughly, give us the gospel on juicing, Gershon therapy, apricot kernels, heat therapy, reiki and any other number of alternative medicine cures or preventions. It takes no more than two minutes of internet research to demonstrate that for each of these treatments there is, at the very least, controversy or disagreement about their efficacy. Case not proven.

Failing to reveal this to readers of your cancer book ought to raise questions about the integrity of the author. But it should also make readers question whether anything else in the book is true. Some of it might indeed be sound science. But if they've failed to properly research or share even the basics, then why should a reader rely on anything else in the book? Particularly when it is our health they're claiming to be an expert in.

Another way to discover if someone is an expert or not is to ask whether they have achieved a particular academic credit for their craft, from a real university or a respected governing body. The terms 'homeopath', 'naturepath', 'life coach', 'nutritionist', 'health coach' and many others like them are not protected terms. I could put a sign outside my door today and call myself a 'homeopath' and need not have mixed a potion in my life. Alternative medicine practitioners are trading on names like these, or 'qualifications' from governing bodies set up and governed by other practitioners using similarly unprotected and invented titles. The certificates and letters of commendation they award to each other do not mean a thing.

If your trained medical doctor messes up, gives you bad advice, or treats you poorly, you have legal recourse. In the UK, you can complain through the NHS or the General Medical Council. In the USA, you can complain to your state's medical council. If upheld, your doctor could be struck off and no longer able to practise medicine. You could get a substantial payout too. In the alternative medicine world, there is no such governing body. There is no 'striking off' because you can't remove an invented title like 'nutritionist', nor can you prevent someone practising. You have no legal recourse to someone giving you bad homeopathic advice. Medical doctors have legal procedures, requirements, training and processes to ensure they're giving you the best treatment the science has proven. Alternative medicine gives you none of this.

I'm not a doctor. I do have a degree but it is not in medical science. I do have a brain tumour. Like the scientific process, I'm as interested in the things I've got wrong as in the things I've got right. I'd love to hear logical responses to my arguments. As long as you're nice about it. But I'm not an expert. And I'll never claim to be.

When I used to work as a copywriter for charities, my colleagues and I did a lot of work for the charity Macmillan Cancer Support. Our role was straightforward enough: to turn sometimes complex and inaccessible cancer information into more simple, more reassuring language that got the messages across the best way we could. We tried to be patient-centred, to put ourselves in the shoes of the people reading our words for the first time.

I always admired the organisation, and it was highly regarded in the sector as the act most other charities wanted to follow: people-focused, great information, great services, incredible communications. Of course, I never expected to be on the receiving end of their work.

Today I am at the organisation not as a writer but − as we used to call them − a 'service user'. I'm in the Macmillan Cancer Centre, part of London's University College Hospital. It's a multi-million pound partnership between the two, with other charitable funders.

One day all hospitals will be like this. As I walk through the revolving door, I'm greeted by a smiling, clipboard wielding welcomer. She asks me how she can help me, and I tell her I'm here to see my oncologist. She directs me to an automatic check-in machine under which I can scan the barcode on my appointment letter. My welcomer, who I discover is a volunteer, invites me to take a seat in the spacious, beautifully designed modern waiting lobby. These are comfy chairs. Almost sofas. In one corner there is a Costa Coffee bar with free WiFi. In another, a huge Macmillan Cancer Support information library. High above my head there's a colourful art installation and gigantic paintings on the walls. Most walls are modern glass panelling, with toilets and entrances hidden flush against them. Dotted around the place are screens, every now and again flashing up a patient's name, directing them where to go next.

I wait for 15 minutes in a chair so comfortable I almost fall asleep. Then a gentle reassuring tone sounds and my name flashes up directing me to a new waiting area. The whole centre has the atmosphere of somewhere to come and relax before your appointment, not to get anxious and disgruntled that your appointment time has run over. From the moment you walk through the door, there's the impression that the charity and hospital have consulted with people who have cancer about every element, every process and colour. What will reduce stress? What might provide reassurance? What might make things more comfortable and convenient if you have to wait in the hospital regularly?

Because in public hospitals, you do have to wait. That's part of the deal. If I have to wait for appointments and treatments over the coming months, I'm glad it's here that I'll do it. In fact, the meeting with my oncologist is a full two hours late. I barely notice the time going by.

My oncologist is friendly and efficient, and she cuts right to the information I've come here for. My tumour does have the 1p/19q and the IDH1 'deletions'. This means the radiotherapy and chemotherapy I'll need to have will be more successful at attacking the cancer. It means my life expectancy is likely to be longer than it would have been.

Then she begins to outline my treatment plan. I'm to have six weeks of radiotherapy every day, except for weekends. The radiographers will mould a plastic mask onto my face, which I'll have to have screwed over my head each day while the radiotherapy is beamed into my brain. Once that's done, I'll have six cycles of chemotherapy, and each of those cycles will be six weeks long. I'll come in once per cycle for an intravenous dose, then take the rest of the drugs at home. She hands me a package of information about the treatments, a full booklet about the side effects I might expect.

I do the sums in my head. Six weeks, plus six times six

weeks. I'm going to be in treatment for 42 weeks, and that's only if things go smoothly. Just shy of a year. It's May. The sun is shining outside.

"There's no particular rush," she says.

These are the words I have been hoping for. Just how desperate is starting treatment now, rather than delaying it for a while to enjoy one last summer before it kicks in? Particularly now my seizures have fallen into a more stable pattern.

Since leaving the meeting with my brain surgeon, I've had the inkling of an idea that waiting to start treatment may be better than beginning it right away. But only if my oncologist thinks that's sensible. My surgeon had said the medical team disagreed about whether to treat my tumour as a grade II or a grade III, so there is at least one indication that there might be no rush. My surgeon had even said some of the medical team didn't think it was clear enough to encourage immediate treatment. I've also looked at the medical papers. It's not clear from the medical literature whether having early treatment – if the tumour can't be operated on – makes much difference in terms of life expectancy. And not knowing my life expectancy, it's still not clear what 'early' and 'later' even means.

But there's something else. If there's no particular rush, I'd rather spend the summer when my kids will be off school with them. My little boy will start pre-school at the end of the summer. I'd rather be enjoying the cycling and the sun while the weather is good, than having treatment, experiencing any side effects and being away from my family.

I realise I'm in an extremely privileged position to even consider this. I don't want to be flippant. It's not easy. Many with cancer don't get close to a choice about when to have treatment. Their life is mapped out. It's like they're on a conveyor belt; restrictive and impersonal. But we get mixed up about choice. We think it entitles us to consider any treatment, rather than those that will actually work for us. My choice is one made within the boundaries of the rationally available options.

I explain my thoughts to my oncologist, and she simply nods, smiles and hands over the information she's gathered.

"I'm entirely comfortable with that," she says. And she means it. We'll wait for my next MRI scan, due towards the end of the summer. If my vascularity has continued to increase and the tumour has shown signs of abnormal growth or malignancy, we'll know for sure. Then we'll plan for treatment starting in the autumn. It feels like she's relieved. She's not desperate to get me under the machine, or to pump chemo into my veins. Her medical opinion is that it's best to wait, if that's what I want to do. I decide that it is. I pledge to her that when it is her professional opinion to put me into cancer treatment, I'll be right there ready to take it. I feel fitter and healthier than I have done for some time. And a decision rationally made with professional, informed, advice is empowering.

Time to talk

SIX MONTHS CAN roll around so quickly, especially when the sun is shining. It's been half a year since my biopsy. Almost as long since my oncologist and I agreed we'd wait until after the summer to begin the radiotherapy and chemotherapy she had planned.

I'm sitting in my neurologist's waiting room again, alongside the other brain tumour patients. This time I have no nerves. This appointment is a necessary routine. We already know what's coming: growth in the tumour, growth in the vascularity, and another pass to my oncologist to start treatment as agreed. But if the tumour does show an increase in vascularity or growth, outwardly I'm showing no signs of it. I'm now going many days at a time without seizures.

The summer has been a good one. I've put in some serious miles on the bike, taken in Alpine climbs and put down some not embarrassing times in the process. I've even raced my bike, something I never thought I'd do again. There have been glorious warm days with my children and friends. A wonderful final summer before life-changing treatment will begin. It's what I wanted.

I do not know – because no one can tell me – how long I have to live. I do not know how long treatment may extend my life. I don't even know the extent of the side effects that may result from the radiotherapy and chemotherapy. I can only put my life in the hands of people I have come to trust: my medical team who know far more about my brain tumour than I do. They set the boundaries between which I can make decisions. That's the rational way to behave, and I understand that they know best.

In my hands I carry the summary of a scientific paper written about blood vascularity in brain tumours. It analysed a group of low-grade tumour patients, measuring their tumour's base vascularity at the start of the study. It then looked at when the patient's tumour transformed from grade II into grade III. It concluded the tipping point for low-grade tumours turning into higher-grade ones was when a patient had a base vascularity of above 1.75. In other words, of all those who had a vascularity lower than 1.75 when they entered the study, only half had transformed into high-grade tumours a full 12 years later. Of those who had a base vascularity above 1.75, half of them had tumours that transformed into high grade just eight months later. My tumour's vascularity was measured at the beginning of this year. It was 4.8.

I'm also holding a 2008 study written by my own neurologist. It looked at the rate of change in the vascularity in tumours over a period of 36 months. It concluded that when patients' vascularity hardly changed from MRI to MRI, their tumour didn't transform into a higher grade during the period of the study. But when the vascularity increased from MRI to MRI, it was a strong indicator that transformation had or was about to take place. In fact, the paper concluded, this increase in vascularity was a far stronger predictor of transformation than a tumour's growth, the side effects it creates or its intensity on the MRI images. So even if the tumour isn't growing or if your seizures aren't getting worse, if your vascularity is increasing there's a good chance transformation is underway. My 4.8 vascularity test was a significant increase on the one before.

It's why I'm sitting here in the waiting room feeling calm. I already know what's going to happen today. I may have made hay while the sun shines this summer, but now it has come to an end. I'm ready to start treatment.

My neurologist greets me in his normal way: his eyes searching for familiarity, trying to put my name and my case together. He finally places me, sits my wife and me down and pulls up my latest MRI scans on his computer. There are two medical students in the corner, taking notes. My neurologist scrolls through my scans, up and down like last time, comparing my latest with the ones that have gone before.

"No," he says matter-of-factly. "All looks stable here, no growth outside of what we'd normally expect from a low-grade glioma." It's as if he's forgotten all about the vascularity, the biopsy, the seizures, everything. I remind him. It's rude, but I highlight his paper on vascularity. Shouldn't I, on his figures, be in the danger zone here?

He gives me his disarming smile. "Let's see, vascularity," He turns back to his computer. This time the perfusion scan has come in.

"Ah, your results are actually lower than they were last time. Your vascularity has gone down. What can I say? You're an oddball."

He looks puzzled in his chair, staring again at my MRIs. "In fact, I don't think I've ever seen this in a brain tumour like yours."

"So surely that means something," I say.

"On the contrary," he says. "It means exactly nothing. No growth is no growth." His scientific paper doesn't quite concur with what he's saying, but I'm off the scale anyway because my vascularity has reduced, not risen. I'm an outlier.

"So, what do you want to do?" he says.

"Well, I guess nothing."

"Good, that sounds like a plan."

In those words, he's swept away any need for radiotherapy or chemotherapy anytime soon. I don't need to see my oncologist. I'm still grade II, and that's how he intends to continue for now. I'm dazed but delighted to agree with him. He turns to the medical students: "You should read his blog, he's a professional cyclist."

I'm not a professional cyclist. I'm nothing even close. But I don't correct him.

"Good," he says to me. He shakes mine and my wife's hands. He gives me a date for another MRI in six months' time. He shows us out and is again speaking into his dictaphone before we've even left the room. My wife and I go for coffee. The usual routine.

The first 18 months of the last years of my life are over. The tumour, of course, continues to grow. Stable doesn't mean doing nothing. It means doing what slow-growing tumours do. Slowly growing. Change is inevitable. The question is always: how much change? I used to think that at these results meetings, no news was good news. I now know it really means: it could always be worse. But there's no malignancy as yet, and the growth is not yet so significant as to affect me any more than seizures and occasional language confusion.

Are we having a grown-up and open conversation about cancer, its treatments and alternative approaches? Are we even talking properly about not having treatments and about dying?

I can't speak for other countries, but in the UK we seem to be lacking a clear narrative about what cancer means to us as individuals and as a community, and how we as a nation should respond.

Our problem perhaps is a mix of politics, money, the behaviour of doctors and alternative medicine practitioners, and the overtly emotional reaction we have to cancer as patients and families.

This whole tendency can be illustrated by the fraught story of Ashya King, a five-year-old boy with a medulloblastoma brain tumour who was receiving treatment in a hospital in Southampton, UK. His parents, unwilling to accept that the treatments on offer to him were the most appropriate for his condition, took their son out of the hospital. They eventually ended up in Spain.

They wanted him to undergo proton-beam therapy, a more modern version of radiotherapy that is not available in the UK for his condition. It's not available because, for his condition, it is no more effective than regular radiotherapy. His family were unwilling to accept this, so took him away. Fearing for for their son's health – he needed very specialist care – the hospital called in British police to track the family down. For a very short time his parents were arrested by Spanish police, who were acting according to their own procedures rather than under instruction from British officers.

Most of the British newspapers went wild, calling the family's treatment barbaric. The British public jammed the Southampton hospital switchboard calling the staff there all kinds of names. Social media went crazy with threats against the doctors – including death threats – because they had refused the boy the treatment his parents had wanted. British politicians, including the Prime Minister, David Cameron, called for the family to be reunited.

The 'manhunt' topped the British news agenda for days. Eventually, the NHS relented and paid for him to undergo the treatment in the Czech Republic because by that time the family had gone there anyway. But at no point did the NHS doctors say his treatment was likely to be any more successful than what they'd recommended for him in the first place.

In the heat of those few days, much was said between parties, verbal punches were thrown, and many thousands of people who had no idea at all what the real issues were waded in. A calmer retrospective look at what happened is very revealing about some of the major issues we're failing to deal with as a society.

First is the idea that the 'parents know best' about what's most favourable for their child. As instinctively true as this may seem to us, when it comes to most medical situations it's just not so. And it's dangerous to assume it is. The King's little boy was surrounded by an expert brain tumour team in Southampton, who were trying to tell the family what treatment would offer their son the best chances of survival. They also offered them a second opinion from other doctors – though an independent review of the case highlighted that their delay in organising one was perceived as a brush off by the family.

Nevertheless, the family had spent a few days on the internet, decided proton-beam therapy was best for their son, and taken him away from the hospital because the oncologists didn't concur with what they'd found online. Armed only with franticly obtained information from the internet, the family had been wrong.

Later, the family started posting YouTube videos of him, along with the feeding machine they had taken from the hospital and the food they had obtained, to show they knew what they were doing to look after him. They didn't. They had not received treatment on how to use the machine nor how to prepare the equipment in a sterile way, according to the independent review. What if their son had taken a turn for the worse or gone into epileptic seizures? How were they protecting his lungs from infection from the feeding tube? In their son's fragile state, he was extremely susceptible to infections that even hospital intensive care units have a battle to control. The parents did not know better. The trained and accountable hospital, its doctors and nurses, did.

Perhaps too there was a breakdown in communication, no

doubt thanks to the fraught circumstances of a little boy's health. Perhaps the family misunderstood what doctors were saying. The prevailing opinion seemed to be that it was all about money: doctors and the NHS weren't willing to pay for the expensive proton-beam therapy his parents wanted. And that's certainly how some newspapers reported it. But that wasn't the case at all. Proton-beam is more expensive but the NHS does pay for it for those for whom it is the best treatment, including for children. In this case, it wasn't appropriate. Money didn't come into it.

And then there was the role played by the newspapers, fuelled again by lack of information and proper communication. This was now a story of a poor oppressed family with a dying five-year-old, on the run from a hospital who had turned them in to the police. Without fully understanding the issues, the British public took their lead from the media and waded in with their own opinions and judgements, leading to abuse of the doctors and the NHS as a whole. Ever conscious of their PR profile, the politicians couldn't help but get involved too.

The independent review concluded that the doctors did not do anything wrong in the King case, except for not anticipating the media interest in the case. The vacuum of information left by the doctor's failure to communicate with the media, it concluded, was dangerous because it might have lead to other children with serious medical issues being taken away from hospitals by parents who did not have the expertise that doctors have.

Politics. Money. Media. Communication. Emotion. It was an unholy mess that could have been avoided if we all had a better knowledge about cancer and took a more rational approach to all of the issues it can involve.

The failure of conventional doctors and alternative medicine practitioners to communicate with each other is likely to present a very real problem for us as we take on cancer into the future. In the British *Guardian* newspaper, Dr Ranjana Srivastava reflects on her frustration that many doctors and alternative medicine practitioners don't talk to each other. She questions whether doctors are so dismissive of alternative medicine that they won't consider the possibility that talking to patients about any alternative medicine they're undergoing might lead to better outcomes. Meanwhile, alternative medicine practitioners are too dismissive of the mainstream cancer establishment to talk to medical doctors.

It puts patients in the ludicrous position of being treated at the same time by two entirely separate individuals or teams of people who don't have anything to do with each other. Most frequently, they don't even know of each other's role with the patient. She writes, "I honestly don't consider arrogance a good explanation for why oncologists and alternative practitioners don't talk. I would, however, say that dismay and distrust feature heavily."

Often, the ugly mudslinging between mainstream and alternative medicine does nothing to open up these conversations, nor each other's understanding of their methods or intentions. Better communication could highlight to the conventional doctor the very real risk of conflicting treatments – chemo drugs and herbal remedies, for example – actually making a patient worse. The conventional doctor could argue her case with the alternative practitioner about why a patient should go for conventional treatment and ensure there are no harms being caused by alternative therapies.

My understanding is that a few doctors and alternative medicine practitioners are communicating better that they have been. Some medical doctors are at least trying to understand *why* patients or their children are pursuing an alternative medicine regime. Instead of dismissing them as irrelevant or 'woo', or simply ignoring the alternative treatment altogether, they're using it as an entry point to address the patients underlying fears and misunderstandings about conventional medicine. They're at least working with their eyes open, and they're working *with* the patient as an individual. They're using what they've got, to try to bring the patient round to what is likely to be best for them. The result can only be better care. But it is clear these doctors are the exception, rather than the rule.

In the same way, the same lack of communication prevents alternative medicine from understanding the real and most up-to-date nature of modern conventional medicine, and the most modern treatments for cancer. It has come an awful long way in the last decade. The old accusation of 'cut, poison, burn' is horribly outdated, replaced most often now by powerful, tailored drugs and gene-based treatments.

There might even be something conventional medicine *can* learn from alternative medicine, if only conversations could happen and together the practitioners could try to pin down what about the alternative treatment seemed to be working for the patient. That could then be followed up through rigorous research. More alternative medicine might just end up becoming conventional medicine after all.

But mostly doctors and alternative medicine practitioners are not talking to each other. Patients are not talking to each other. And no one, with a very few exceptions, is having a grown up conversation about any of this. We as cancer patients, others as the world's future cancer patients, and we as humans trying to live together as best we can in the face of the disease can only come out all the worse.

We talk of cancer being all about patient choice but this failure to talk among practitioners of either hue is actually curtailing choice and knowledge. Doctors may feel they don't have the time to waste talking to 'quacks', but in the long term if it saves more lives or stops doctors from having to pick up the pieces when alternative medicine has created a mess, isn't that something they should at least consider?

In the same way, what is really missing among both medical and alternative practitioners, and among patients, families, politicians and the media too, is a sensible conversation about our approach to dying. And particularly about dying from cancer.

In the NHS there is certainly an attitude that patients with cancer must be kept alive for as long as possible, at any cost. I'm talking here about those with terminal cancer, where treatment is aimed at keeping a patient alive for a month or two longer, rather than those being treated because they might be cured or their life could be extended for a considerable amount of time. Many expensive, painful and quality-of-life-reducing treatments, including radiotherapy, chemotherapy and surgery, are being applied again and again to the same patients to give them an extra month or two each time.

This happens perhaps because patients themselves, and their family, don't want to let go. Any extra time, they believe, even if it is of poor quality is better than no time at all. It also perhaps happens because a doctor feels their obligation is to keep even very sick people alive. There's an innate contradiction in the hippocratic oath doctors adhere to, which charges them to preserve life but also to prevent suffering. So they keep going back to the same terminally ill patient because the alternative is to willingly let them die.

Our attitude to dying from cancer brings this into relief. A discussion about a patient's preferences, or a discussion with patients and families about a doctor's realistic abilities and role, rarely takes place.

There is a case to be made that such conversations should take place earlier in a person's cancer journey. Even, perhaps, if a patient's chances of survival are quite high. There should be a cultural shift where talking about chances of death and what should happen if the worst is on the cards becomes the norm. Because it's a much more difficult conversation to have when something needs to be done in an emergency, when everything is frantic, when everyone is grieving and under pressure to make radical, literally life-changing decisions.

My brother was so confused about his own illness, he never even realised he had cancer until he started turning up for radiotherapy and noticed many fellow patients spent so much time talking about it. Not for a second did he think he might not live through it. No one had ever talked to him about his illness in those terms, even though not surviving was certainly a possibility. I hope my own ignorance of the seriousness of his condition is to blame for my treating it in such a blasé way at the time.

Cancer, I have discovered, is all about questions: what about this treatment? Should I start this diet? How long have I got? The question we're mostly failing to address is: what should we do when the end of life is inevitable? Should we keep pushing through invasive and uncomfortable treatment for every extra month we can squeeze out? When should we choose to move to palliative care? What is the threshold that needs to be passed?

In my case, I hated the idea that doctors would be forced through lack of knowledge of my preferences to keep me alive through repeating treatment after treatment to gain little slivers of extra time. I felt it wouldn't be how I'd want to exit this earth. It's not something I want my family to have to suffer, let alone leave my wife to have to make a decision about. And it's not something I want doctors to have to decide for themselves when they have more hopeful cases to attend to.

As a result, I wrote what in the UK we call an 'Advanced Decision'. It's a legal document that outlines the lengths I will allow doctors to go to in order to keep me alive. Given what I've written so far, you won't be surprised to learn that once the end is relatively imminent I'd err on the side of non-intervention. Make me comfortable, prop me up in front of the cycling on the TV and let me go. I certainly don't want doctors to eke out my life, particularly if that life is likely to be of lower quality than if they just leave me to it.

These are conversations I'm sure many of us have had in the pub, or with our partners, or late into the night when talking with friends. But rarely do we actually have these conversations with our doctors, leaving them to have to make difficult decisions on our behalf, or worse perhaps to oblige them to keep intervening when really we'd rather have been left to die.

If we had these conversations with our oncologists, we could have discussions that were better informed, and then write better Advanced Decisions or their equivalent, because we'd know what our deaths were likely to look like.

Interestingly – though let's be clear that this is from a single clinical study, so should be treated with some caution – one study from Lille in France revealed that those who opted for a structured, well-funded end-of-life plan for their final months of cancer, tended to actually live longer than those who insisted on every intervention to try to keep them alive. And planned palliative care certainly led to better quality of life than the 'give it all you've got' alternative.

Inevitably, and unfortunately, the spectre of money and politics also comes into this. That study showed, for example, that the quality palliative care that tended to lead to a longer life also cost far less than the continual intervention approach. In countries like the USA where people are expected to pay health insurance to cover their risk of cancer, there are very significant implications: will health insurance companies begin dictating an end-of-life plan for us because it is cheaper than the alternative? Will they refuse to fund the continual intervention approach at all?

In the UK, the implications are more societal than business or profit orientated. The NHS is a free-at-the-point-of-need service. We pay for the NHS in our taxes, and in most cases don't pay again for any health interventions we have throughout our lives. It's already been clearly shown that the continual intervention approach to one person's life uses enough resources (essentially money) in the NHS that, if it were applied elsewhere, could save many more lives.

I'm not for a second suggesting our desire to cling to life is selfish, or that we should make decisions about our own life length by weighing it up against the lives of others. That's too far a leap to make and too big a burden to lay at the feet of cancer patients.

But we do have to recognise, and often fail to do so, that these are decisions that politicians and those at the head of health services (and indeed insurance companies) have to make. It's too much to expect them to make decisions on a case-by-case basis, though sometimes they may feel pressured into doing so. But they do certainly have to draw up the policies by which these issues are decided. Politicians and heads of health services are always talking about tough decisions, and these decisions must be some of the hardest. We elect (or pay) people to make these decisions for us, and I don't envy them.

But we can help by joining them in the debate and informing their decision-making by properly understanding the issues at stake, and communicating amongst ourselves, with our doctors, politicians and other decision makers about the nature of cancer and dying. It's the conclusion I've come to again and again when writing my thoughts about cancer. Where possible we need to discuss cancer and dying without getting overly caught up in emotion. And that means those who are not, or not yet, intimately involved with the disease need to talk alongside those of us who are actually affected by the decisions at stake.

And perhaps the very first, most difficult, opening question in the whole debate, but one which is almost unutterable in our society, is this: when does death become acceptable?

At time of writing, I am 38 years old. By most people's standards, my death from cancer would be considered tragically young. But at what point does my death become more acceptable? 48? 68? 88?

Death is never acceptable in terms of something to be welcomed, happy about, celebrated. At least not in the traditional sense. Death is horrible and it hurts those left behind. But at what age, or in what circumstances, or with what quality of life, do we as a society say: well, that's about right, isn't it?

You may feel I'm playing a numbers game here and it is true that the key cause of the increase in cancer prevalence in the western world is down to us all living longer. But the question is valid nevertheless. We're outraged by a child's death from cancer, but we seem less outraged when it is an 88-year-old. So somewhere, unarticulated perhaps, we do have some kind of societal moral imperative about what is an acceptable age to reach. Does the unacceptability of death lessen for every year we manage to live?

Perhaps more importantly, at what age does death come without blame? When a child dies, or a cancer patient doesn't get the treatment they wanted or thought was best for them, we are quick to lay blame at someone's feet. If only doctors had done this, or diagnosed earlier, or not attempted surgery or allowed chemotherapy, they'd still be alive. Death is hard to accept and it's natural to look for someone to blame. But at what stage do we stop looking for someone to release that emotion upon? At what point do we accept that death is just the way it goes?

I'm as confused as everyone else about these conflicting emotions. It would be a very bold politician or hospital manager indeed who drew a line in the sand and said, say, 85 is the tipping-point age. Or decided that when your quality of life, or physical or mental abilities, have deteriorated past a certain non-returnable point, that the line for 'worthwhile life' has been crossed.

But again, for the most part we're still not having this conversation. There's a taboo and it hampers a rational discussion about cancer, about its treatments, their effectiveness and the alternatives on offer. And it leads to some ludicrous conclusions.

If, for example, I am receiving some mainstream cancer prevention strategy, or following an alternative cancer prevention diet, at what age am I entitled to conclude: well, that worked! We did it! I've successfully prevented cancer. Don't we end up in the strange position of doing everything we can to stave off cancer in order for us to die from something else? What kind of success is that? Preventing cancer long enough to develop heart failure, or dementia, or to trip and bang our heads because our bones and muscles are so frail becomes some kind of victory?

Whether undergoing conventional treatment, or alternative interventions, our general lack of communication about what we really mean by cure, living, death, an acceptable death or even a good death, means we can only muddle along hoping for the best.

This is where my brain tumour story ends for now. My physical and medical life has taken on an almost predictable pattern. I feel ill for a while, a few weeks where I have to sleep a lot, I can never get my head straight, there's a constant weakness in my right-hand side, and the seizures are far deeper, affect my language and are prone to take place at any time. Then for a few weeks, I feel relatively normal. I'm fit, sociable and happy. I have many seizures every day – more frequently than during the bad weeks – but they're very light, passing almost beyond notice. I take care of my kids. I cycle a lot, sometimes I even race. My little boy has started big school. I'm working as a writer. Life has gone on when once I thought it had already finished.

I am a member of the six-month club. I go for my half-yearly scans, and each one still feels like it could be the harbinger of bad news. One day it will be, but right now it's only news of a slow growth. Daily, I still take a full handful of drugs. I've now admitted my seizures will never go away. I'll never drive again. But for the time being, this is my life and my life is continuing.

But that does not mean I am normal in my mind. The diagnosis flipped a minor and occasional dissatisfaction with my professional life into something much deeper. Looking over my planning diary for the last three years, I see entry after entry, urging me: 'brainstorm career options', 'make a plan', 'decide what you want to do with your life', 'make final decisions', 'this time, finally, finally decide on your future…'

When I have finished writing the words you've been reading, I know I'll enter similar entries in my diary for the months to come. Today, I have an idea of retraining to become a teacher. On the weekend I was discussing setting up a bike-come-coffee shop. There's also that novel I want to write. Indecision is not something unique to those with a brain tumour. The oscillating waves between fantasy, practicality, effort and possibility are not something particular only to those with a life limiting disease. But I feel it acutely. As a member of the six-month club, there are restrictions on my opportunities to really decide who I am.

And also I feel guilt. Guilt mainly for being still alive, when others with brain tumours diagnosed since mine have already passed away. In 1772, the German composer Joseph Haydn wrote a symphony called *The Farewell*. At the end, each member of the orchestra one by one stops playing, packs up their music and leaves the stage. The number of musicians dwindles until only a single violinist remains to conclude the piece and turn out the lights. The theme was picked up by the celebrated novelist Edmund White in his semi-autobiographical novel of the same name. He was writing about the AIDS crisis in New York during the 1980s. His protagonist is forced to watch each of his friends on the gay scene die, and his friendship group dwindles to no more than just a handful. Like him, I feel guilt at being lucky enough to carry on playing.

I feel guilt too when I see my friends who, at the beginning, rallied around my family with their love and sympathy, their support financial and physical. I feel like a fraud when I look at them and I'm still fit and healthy, and the only answer I can answer to the question of "how are you?" is, "Same as usual." I'm a fraud, reaping the rewards then failing to repay them with my decline.

The best prediction of my life expectancy I've ever received, from the medical literature, is a median around 14 years. That means half the people with my condition will die before that, half after. I'm embarrassed to offer this number when a radio interviewer asked me about my prognosis. He'd introduced me as having terminal cancer. Fourteen years doesn't sound very terminal, does it? It's almost another half the life I've already lived. This is not what I promised when it was originally diagnosed and asked for sympathy. It's not what our original panic justified. Then I feel further guilt because I know that not for a second do my friends think this way. That even my thinking that of them is selfish and mean.

But even as I write those words, I am reminded that I am worried about the future. About my life, my treatment, and the family I will eventually leave behind. I have to pinch myself and stay in the present because what will be will be. I don't mean that life has a plan for me, or even what I know now about my condition will not change as progress and research takes brain tumour survival on slowly longer trajectories. All I know is that whatever journey it takes, my life will no longer look like it does now. And I know that whatever twists and turns that journey takes, scientific research and medical discovery will help to steer the path.

Looking back now with the 'better end of the bad ones', I'm sure that the first year of panic my wife and I lived was misguided and perhaps unnecessary. I now know that clinicians and doctors and nurses were trying to tell us that at the time. But the panic and the fear, the crumbling and the chaos was real nevertheless. When I told the Brain Tumour Charity's fundraising video cameras we were worried whether I'd even see my son start school, it wasn't a cynical play for sympathy and money. I really did think I was already on my way out.

Both of our children are now at school. They're well, and they both understand that I am well for now. They know that Daddy has a brain tumour, which is a type of cancer and that cancer is not good. They know it causes me to have 'dizzies' and sometimes to be very tired and unwell. They know it will never go away, and one day it will make me very ill. They tell me they will look after me. Erin says she wants to take out my poorly brain through the hole the biopsy left, then fill my head with strawberries.

However well we pretended in that first year that we were OK, however we tried to put on a sheen of dealing with it rationally and philosophically, we both now understand that there was always deep swell raging just under the calmer surface. With patients of dementia who have become convinced thanks to their disease they are still living in the

1950s, it can be confusing and even unnerving to keep telling them they are wrong. It was the same for us. Some, perhaps most, of our friends and our doctors could see the world we had built around ourselves. And they gracefully kept their peace, allowing us to deal with my diagnosis in the way that worked best for us.

Now I feel different. Perhaps I am continuing to kid myself. Perhaps underneath my calm acceptance life remains the swirl of torment. But I don't think so. Now, I think, we know where we have been and where we are going. That doesn't mean it's not scary, or that we are unrealistic about what is to come. The truth is still there. I have an appointment card with an MRI scan on it that reminds me every time I forget. But sometimes, more often than before, I wake up in the mornings and the tumour isn't the first thing I think about.

Cancer never goes away, even if you're declared 'clear'. Over time my brain tumour and its symptoms have faded in significance and life has taken on a kind of newly-drawn normality. I can't live in a panic every day as we wait for the worst to happen. The sun will still rise tomorrow whether I feel good or bad.

Hope

OTHER CANCER BOOKS have bright covers, sunsets and colourful fruits and vegetables (inevitably on their way to be juiced), shining ribbons and smiling faces. They urge you to be determined to 'beat' or 'fight' or 'accept' or 'embrace'. In this company, there will be readers who accuse me of being devoid of hope, and in cancer circles 'hope' is chanted like a mantra without which you are doomed to not even wanting to live. Perhaps you even deserve to lose your battle against cancer.

If you think I am devoid of hope, then you are wrong. But perhaps it is not quite the same meaning of 'hope' that you assume. I do desperately want to live and I hope to live as long as possible, perhaps even to 70 or 80 or whatever age society deems acceptable and proper. But my hope is one centred in realism and rationalism.

I cannot and will not hope that my tumour will magically shrink and go away. My brother's cancer was thankfully completely cured by chemo and radiotherapy. He barely thinks of it today, though for a year of his life it was the only thing on his and his wife's mind. But I cannot hope for the same eventual outcome.

Why hope for the impossible? There is no current scientific research that makes such a promise, and nor any serious predictions that such a cure is even on the horizon. But within the science that does currently exist, and within the biological possibility now tentatively suggested, there is the possibility – the hope – of extending my life. A hope that could become a reality. It's a hope justified by knowledge, not magic or wishful thinking.

There are techniques: genetically targeted medication, immune-based therapies, improved radiotherapy, better imaging and perhaps even better surgical methods, that month after month, year after year, are slowly but surely improving. They are being tested, proven and then becoming mainstream. But there's no magic fix. For every development there are a dozen dead ends and blind corners, a hundred disappointments. These things take time, but perhaps I am lucky. Having a low-grade brain tumour means that time is most likely to be on my side. The longer I manage to live, the more scientific progress is likely to be made to treat my illness.

There is a chance that I'll live long enough for this science to become applicable to me. A chance that the medical research will one day mean the treatment stays one step ahead of my tumour, rather than my tumour staying one step ahead of the treatment. And if cancer can be kept at bay for the rest of my life (noting of course the strange philosophical problem such a concept entails) then what's the difference between having cancer or not? I don't want to live forever, but I do want a fair shot at it.

But in the meantime, science moves slowly. It can't be rushed, and that's necessary and important. Most medical trials aren't about curing particular patients, they're about little cells in petri dishes, and perhaps this is something that needs to be made clearer to those offered a chance to participate. Most clinical trials are studies involving large numbers of people. They are, by necessity, the opposite of individual treatment. To participate in science only to benefit myself would be selfish and to believe it could cure me is on the verge of misguided. But as long as I'm in this tricky situation, I believe I have a responsibility to contribute to the wider search for a cancer cure. Maybe I can be a little brick in the tower that will eventually break through. It gives me heart and makes me proud to be able be part of that. It is a shame that so many who choose unproven, unrealistic alternative medicine and experimental treatments, without any monitoring whatsoever, don't see the value of these slowly building blocks towards a cure. It's a shame they can't see that if they participated in a properly regulated, peer-reviewed trial, their own experience could contribute to the wider good too.

Whatever life I've lived, and whatever life awaits me, I hope it is life based on honesty and enquiry, on wonder at the complexity, yet nevertheless explainability of the world. I don't want to live a lie, based on pretending or a miraculous kind of hope. I want my children to understand and believe in science, to see its amazing and awesome possibility, but also its current limitations. That's the price you pay for truth. Much better to be honest, however harsh and cruel. To understand that life sometimes is devoid of hope and miraculous endings, than to believe in magic. For my children, hocus pocus may soften the initial blows but wouldn't it make the reality all the more painful when the masquerade is revealed?

These are just the thoughts of a young man. A man who has faced challenges trying to come to understand and to come to terms with his life-limiting disease. But I hope I'm a man who, despite the tumour in his brain, has a clear and rational mind. Without rational understanding of the world around us, the acceptance of what is real and can be understood, what does it mean to be alive anyway?

The world is amazing. I've tried to spend most of my life with my eyes open, and from the day of diagnosis it's how I've treated every aspect of my illness. It's how I'd like to spend the rest of my life too: however long this deadly lump in my rational brain allows it to last.

So, what can we conclude from all this deep thinking about cancer? I know there will be some readers (and indeed many who don't get as far as actually reading most of what I have written) for whom my words will not resonate at all. Whatever I say about science, and rationality, and alternative medicine, and about the very nature of cancer, there's little that will change their minds. There are those who just know alternative medicine can prevent and cure cancer, or that a family should always try anything in the face of cancer. We all like to have our biases confirmed, not challenged, and for that reason this book will receive short shrift or even condemnation among some.

There will be trolls. I will be called names on the internet. There will be those who leave one star for this book on review websites not in response to the quality of my writing, or the quality of my arguments, or because it made them think, but simply because they reject entirely the possibility that alternative medicine might not be correct. Worse, there will be those who firmly believe I too am in the firm grip of the pharmaceutical companies. Everyone gets paid! I'm not. But they'll say it anyway.

To these readers and non-readers, I cannot say much. We shall have to agree to disagree though I do make at least one promise to you. If you can show me firm, peer-reviewed scientific evidence that your cancer prevention therapy or cure works, I will no longer call it alternative medicine. I'll call it medicine. And if proven to work for my particular brain tumour, I'll be first in line for a dose.

What I'm perhaps more worried about is that people will read what I have written here and will mistake my musings for my being callous and cold. On the surface, what I've written seem occasionally pretty harsh, and if you're currently affected by cancer they'll be pretty tough things to read. But I do not personally blame any cancer patient or their family for taking whatever actions they see fit to take. It is their business, and I have no right to judge your personal actions, just as you have no right to judge mine. My comments are meant to question and to analyse a certain tendency in cancer circles and that's not a personal judgement.

Readers may well take my musings as callous and cold, but that doesn't make them any less true. In my defence, I'd like to argue that it is cancer itself that appears cold. By which I mean indiscriminate, uncaring (literally, cancer does not have the capacity to care) and essentially amoral. To blame me for that would be to shoot the messenger.

As a society, we get extremely emotional about cancer. Cancer is so elevated in our fears that we don't make rational decisions. It's OK for people to seek good news in an uncertain world. But that a certain unproven process or therapy makes us feel better about our cancer is not the same as actually *being* better. I can completely understand and appreciate the first because I'm a patient myself. But that doesn't make the latter any less true.

Of course, we cannot talk about cancer in an emotionless way, however much we would like to. Despite what I've written over the last 70,000 words, if my daughter or son were to get a serious cancer and be told by doctors that there was nothing that could be done to save their life or reduce their suffering, I really do not know what I would do. Would my fatherly instincts override my reasoning brain? Would my desperation override my reasonable acceptance of the truth?

That is what being human is all about, and this balance between emotion and reason is what separates us from other animals. My call here is not for people to be less human about cancer. In fact, it's a call to be more human. A call for us to allow the fullness of unique human capacity to play a role when it comes to serious disease, rather than just our knee-jerk and emotional reactions. We have the amazing capacity for reason and critical thinking, and too often we waste its awesome power when we face the most awful of circumstances.

I guess what I'm arguing is that for too long we've allowed cancer to control us, bearing down on patients as if it is more powerful even than what makes us human: our capacity to think. Our desperate search in the face of cancer is not standing up to the disease, it is submitting to its terrifying, mesmerising charms. But those charms are imagined. Cancer is a biological process no more worthy of special regard, excitement or irrational thinking than other biological processes like digestion, or tooth decay, or flowers opening or bees making honey.

This book about my own desperation and resultant thinking about cancer is an appeal for us not to get carried away. Instead, to take control. It's an appeal to the desperate to consider rationally all their options, to ensure they understand the tried and tested scientific method, before judging which way to leap. And whichever way patients do make a leap, whether into alternative or conventional medicine, it's an appeal to ensure that everything about their cancer, tumours, illness, therapies, diet and whatever else relevant, is recorded in a useful, comparable way and made available to trained conventional medicine specialists in oncology. Only then can all of us trying to understand cancer, ways to prevent it and ways to cure it, make those small steps of progress that are needed to get on top of the disease.

It is an appeal to all of us to think about how we as a society deal with cancer, with disease, and even with death. To encourage us to ask in all elements of our lives and deaths: what is appropriate? What is rational? What is reasonable? And what is human?

CPSIA information can be obtained at www.ICGtesting.com
Printed in the USA
LVOW07s0823151115

462645LV00020B/1070/P